The Lazy Person's Guide!

Exercise

To Gemma

I'll miss you so much

love you

I'll really really miss
you
Nadia

Other titles in this series:

The Lazy Person's Guide!

Exercise

Helen Graham

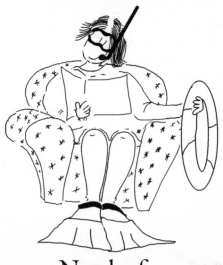

Newleaf

Newleaf

an imprint of
Gill & Macmillan Ltd
Hume Avenue
Park West
Dublin 12
with associated companies throughout the world
www.gillmacmillan.ie

© Helen Graham 2002
0 7171 3302 8
Design by Vermillion Design
Illustration by Emma Eustace
Print origination by Linda Kelly
Printed by ColourBooks Ltd, Dublin

This book is typeset in Rotis Semi-Sans 10pt on 13pt.

The paper used in this book comes from the wood pulp of managed forests. For every tree felled, at least one tree is planted, thereby renewing natural resources.

A CIP catalogue record for this book is available from the British Library.

5 4 3 2 1

CONTENTS

INTRODUCTION

The fact that you've opened this book suggests that you think you are lazy, but you're interested in exercise, if only to the extent of wanting to know more about the conundrum posed by the title. Maybe you think about exercise – you may even like the idea of it – but you don't do anything about it because you can't be bothered. You may have looked at this book in the hope that it offers a quick fix or an effortless remedy: a way to exercise without doing very much. The good news is: *it does.* Furthermore, you're probably not as lazy as you think – for a truly lazy person, reaching out to pick up the book would be overdoing it! So, you're not *totally* lazy and you *are* interested in exercise, at least just a tiny bit. This gives us something to work on.

EXERTION

Let's begin by defining the terms 'lazy' and 'exercise'. What exactly do *you* mean by lazy? Are you comparing yourself to other physically active people – professional sportsmen and women, gymnasts, dancers, those who regularly take part in sport, attend a gym or go jogging, or who are simply on the go all the time? Are you comparing yourself to how physically active you were in the past? Or do you mean that you've always been a couch potato who finds it an effort to work the TV remote? It's most likely that you consider yourself lazy in comparison to how active you think you *should* be.

However you define it, being lazy is always in relation to exercise or exertion. If you're lazy, you're not inclined to exert yourself, but it's unlikely that you never exert yourself in anything – you have, after all, picked up this book and read this far ... You're more likely to be selectively lazy, exerting yourself in activities you like but not in others you regard as hard work. For the lazy, this is the defining feature of exercise. The amount of exertion involved is considered excessive and therefore unpleasant. And so you avoid it. But if you enjoy something, you're more likely to do it, however much exertion or work is involved.

Take Anne, for example. Her New Year's resolution was to exercise more, but she hasn't. When asked why, she says, 'Exercise is hard work and needs discipline.' Yet Anne is enthusiastic about swimming and walking, both of which she does regularly. If you point out this paradox, she says, 'Oh, I don't count swimming and walking. They're enjoyable. They give me a buzz.'

So what does Anne mean by exercise? She knows exactly what she means: 'Working out. Going to a gym. Working hard. And that's not appealing.' Why doesn't Anne simply continue to swim and walk regularly and if she wants to increase the amount of exercise she does, swim and walk more often? The answer is simply that she has a specific mindset about what exercise is: it's not just work, but *hard* work, which makes it neither enjoyable nor appealing. Activities she finds easy and enjoyable don't count as exercise.

So this is the first thing to understand about being lazy: it's in the mind, in the way that you regard activities as exertion or enjoyment.

CONFLICT

While you may differ from Anne in not finding swimming or walking either easy or enjoyable, you may be like her in that you think exercise can't mean *any* activity that seems easy and enjoyable. Why then are you interested in exercise at all? If the answer to this question is, 'Well, I'm not really,' why are you kidding yourself by reading this book? Isn't it more likely that you think you *should* exercise? Or, possibly, you really are interested in exercise, but you're in two minds about it. You want to do more of something you don't want to do at all.

When thinking about whether you're lazy or not, there is always going to be some sort of inner conflict, partly because you don't really want to regard yourself, or be regarded by others, as lazy, but also because you (or other people) think you should be doing something that you're not doing. Back to Anne again. She wants to lose weight, maintain the weight loss, and be more fit and healthy. In the past, she has tried to achieve these things by dieting. But Anne loves food and socialising. Much of her social life involves eating and drinking at office, lunch or dinner parties, suppers, barbecues and picnics. So achieving her ideal weight and improving her health involves constant self-denial. She knows that by increasing her level of activity she will burn off calories because this is what happens when she swims and walks more often. She could therefore *enjoy* eating *and* burning calories but she doesn't because she has bought into the idea that exercise means something difficult and unpleasant that must be avoided. So she opts instead for dieting and self-denial. It's usually when her self-control lapses and she stops dieting and gains weight again that she begins to think she should take more exercise, and this fearful thought (she doesn't count swimming and walking, remember?) is normally enough to propel her back to a strict diet.

It's not surprising that Anne thinks this way. Exercise has been linked in the past with slogans such as 'No pain, no gain' and with the idea that you need to feel your muscles 'burn' for it to be effective. For many people these messages reinforce the negative ideas they already have about exercise: it's a pain in every sense of the word. Everywhere we look we're confronted with images of glamorous super-toned men and women. And exercise videos and books by media stars abound, so we know how hard they have worked under the supervision of tough personal trainers to achieve their look. It seems anyone in the media spotlight *must* reveal to the world the details of their exercise regime. Doing so makes them appear heroic. *'Nowadays, every actress and model tells us how terminally lazy they are ... though celebrities all hate it, they still exercise, which makes them different from you and me'* (Jo Phillimore, 'Why we all hate exercise').

The result of all the media hype is that exercise is increasingly equated with glamour, success, stardom, wealth, power and sex appeal, and has therefore become another pressure on our lives, whether we aspire to those ideals, or not.

EXERCISE AND HEALTH

The reality for most of us is that our lifestyles are increasingly sedentary. In the UK less than 85 per cent of us include any physical activity in our work and only 4 in 10 participate regularly in physical activity. This means that the average person uses 500–800 fewer calories each day than they did ten years ago.

Although the emphasis on exercise being good for our image often diverts our attention away from its other benefits, we all know that exercise is good for our health in all kinds of ways.

Let's remind ourselves.

Exercise protects us against heart disease. It increases energy levels, tones muscles, dilates the blood vessels, lowers blood pressure and heart rate. It increases cardiovascular efficiency, aids the metabolism of carbohydrates and fats so that high levels of sugars, fats and cholesterol in the blood are reduced and high-density lipo-proteins, which protect against heart disease, are raised. It therefore reduces susceptibility to heart attack, stroke and other cardiovascular disease.

Exercise improves the functioning of the lungs and circulatory system, tones and strengthens muscle, including heart muscle, and delays the degenerative effects of ageing, and regular weight-bearing exercise can prevent the onset of osteoporosis, which is the thinning and brittleness of bones resulting from loss of mineral content.

Exercise burns calories, helping to prevent conditions related to the presence of excess body fat, such as hypertension, heart disease, diabetes and cancer.

As well as often being a factor in overweight, which in turn can lead to health problems, physical inactivity itself can place stress on the body by allowing unreleased and unexpressed energy to build up. Exercise reduces tension in the muscles by discharging energy and thus reduces susceptibility to stress-related diseases.

Stress is now recognised as underpinning some 75 per cent of all diseases and contributing significantly to the remainder. However, it can be combated – with exercise.

Exercise can provide many stress-busting benefits. When you exercise regularly, you become much more sensitive to your body and better able to recognise muscle tensions and other signs of stress, and so feelings of control increase. This is important because the belief that you can control events reduces your reaction to stressful situations. Exercise also acts as a distraction from stressful circumstances in your life, allowing you to forget, albeit temporarily, the pressures and frustrations that produced your bodily tensions in the first place. So, by giving yourself a break in this way, you find you are able to deal with stress more effectively.

Having taken up exercise, people often perceive situations as less stressful than they did before and physically fit people react less to stress than those who are less fit. Fitness also protects us from illness during stressful times. In people with low levels of fitness, life stress is strongly related to illness but it has little effect on those whose levels of fitness are higher.

As well as helping us deal with stress more successfully, regular exercise produces other psychological benefits, for example, increased self-esteem and self-confidence. And fitness has also been linked to improvements in mental functioning and general well-being, even helping us maintain our mental ability as we age, reducing the risk of conditions such as Alzheimer's disease.

Our mood can be enhanced by exercise because it relieves symptoms of anxiety, depression and fatigue. Mental anxieties create physical tensions and, by dissipating these through exercise, you send cues to your brain that you are less anxious, giving yourself a mental 'time out' while giving your body a break from tension at the same time.

Given the physical and psychological benefits of exercise, it's as near a panacea as you can get – a health inducer, a stress buster *and* a confidence booster.

RELAXATION – THE LAZY PERSON'S KEY TO SUCCESS

'Uhm,' I hear you say, 'but I still can't see myself going to a gym or taking up a sport.' That's understandable. But there is a solution. You don't have to go to a gym at all. In fact, you don't even have to go out. You can exercise in your own home. You'll avoid the insuperable problem of getting yourself out the door and many of the other psychological problems that are attached to exercise. You'll also overcome the problems of not being able to easily leave the home because of dependants, or if you're a single parent who might otherwise have to get a baby-sitter. Contrary to popular belief, you don't need to exert yourself greatly at all in order to exercise effectively. Better still, you can do so lying down or sitting comfortably. It's the lazy person's dream. But it isn't mere fantasy. It can really happen.

Lazy people use up far too much energy through muscle tension created by inactivity and this has physical and psychological effects that make exercise virtually unthinkable, much less do-able. The fundamental problem for the lazy person – that's you – is that you need to reduce your overall levels of tension and increase your mental and physical energy before you can even consider doing any exercise. Only when you have achieved that will you feel energised enough to include exercise in your life.

Relief from tension is achieved by relaxation. This doesn't mean watching television, reading, socialising, or other things you may associate with relaxing. The reason is that these are all *activities*: they involve *doing* something, even if it is just lying there, and doing something requires the use of muscles, and therefore involves muscle tension. Even when you're lounging in front of the television or lying in bed, muscle tension doesn't necessarily diminish and might even increase. Relaxation literally means loosening and is the opposite of tension or tightening. It means not doing *any*thing. This is difficult for most of us to achieve because we are conditioned to think that we should be doing something all the time. 'Just relax' is therefore one of the most difficult things to put into practice. When you are taking it easy and you think you are doing nothing, you are usually doing a great deal.

Relaxation isn't achieved simply by being idle. You may think you're relaxing, but after several hours no significant changes will have occurred in your body and even when you feel relaxed, and appear to be, deep-seated muscle tension may still remain. This may be revealed in the form of tightness in the muscles of the face, jaw and throat, in your eye movements, or in involuntary or localised reflex actions such as wrinkling of the forehead, blinking and swallowing, irregular breathing and startled responses to sudden noise. Your pulse rate may also remain high.

When you're properly relaxed all tension is absent. There are no visible signs of stiffness in your limbs, the muscles of your face are smooth, your eyelids are motionless, your breathing is regular, you don't constantly blink or swallow, reflexes are absent and your pulse rate lowers. Loosening or relaxing your muscles relieves tension and releases the energy bound up in them, invigorating and vitalising your body. In addition to raising energy levels, staying relaxed improves the condition and tone of the body, counteracts stress and illness, and can also promote weight loss resulting from stress-related patterns of eating and drinking. By relieving tension, relaxation reduces anxiety, and this in itself will enhance your well-being.

Relaxation can therefore be considered an approach that 'works out' the body *and* the mind by releasing tension from both. It shares these benefits with more vigorous exercise but achieves them without exertion, as most of the exercises are performed lying or sitting down.

That's why *The Lazy Person's Guide to Exercise* offers you a programme of relaxation exercises based on a wide range of approaches, and all the exercises are standard, well-established, safe and simple techniques. Now you can make the most of being lazy while learning how to relax properly, and in the long run you'll enjoy all the benefits of exercise without that feeling of over-exertion. You may even find that the effects of relaxation – reducing tension and increasing energy – create a desire in you for more strenuous exercise, so the benefits of walking, and even going to the gym, are covered in the last two chapters, with further related exercises to help you on your way.

So why not give it a go? You can't lose!

CHAPTER 1

HAVING A LIE DOWN

A common mistake made by many people who begin to exercise is to believe that quicker and faster means better. In fact slower and gentler exercise is in many respects more beneficial than vigorous activity. A gentle warm-up eases the body into more energetic activity and also decreases the chance of injury. This is true whether applied to a single exercise session or a programme of exercise over time. Without taking time to develop appropriate techniques exercise can be ineffective and risky. So this guide to exercise begins by showing you how to take it easy.

LEARNING TO UNWIND

Tension is commonly described by those who experience it as feeling 'wound up', 'strung out', 'strung up', 'uptight' or being 'at full stretch', all phrases that accurately reflect its effects on the body. Many people acknowledge the need to loosen up, unwind or wind down – to relax and let go of the tension. The problem is that they don't know how. Instinctively many people in this state feel like lying down. Generally, however, they don't, because they're not in the right place at the time or because they tell themselves they've just got to get on. And from past experience they probably feel that if they take that much-needed lie down they won't unwind anyway and may become even more tense and wound up. Nevertheless, having a lie down really *is* the best thing they could do.

Lying down is the basis of traditional and contemporary approaches to exercise that recognise relaxation as a way of letting go of habitual physical and mental tensions that drain energy from mind and body, making activity difficult. Relaxation is the necessary prerequisite to exercise of any kind. It not only energises the body, enabling it to exercise, but also helps the body to do so without undue tension that might result in injury.

YOGA

Relaxation is fundamental to yoga. The classic yoga position for relaxation is the corpse posture or *savasana*. As its name suggests, it involves simply lying down as if dead. Nothing could be easier.

Exercise 1
Being 'dead relaxed': the corpse posture

Prepare for this exercise as you would for a normal lie down: remove your shoes, socks/tights, any tight clothes, spectacles/contact lenses. Don't attempt it with a full stomach, bladder or bowels. Now:

- Lie flat on your back on a hard floor with your feet together.

- Ensure that your shoulder blades, buttocks and legs are in a straight line and are resting evenly on the floor.

- Let your legs and feet roll away from each other.

- Position your arms slightly away from your body so that they are not in contact with it. Turn the hands palm up and slightly inwards, with the fingers curled loosely towards the palm.

- Position your head so that it is in line with your body and there is no contraction or shortening of the neck muscles.

- Close your eyes.

- Allow your body to sink under its own weight so that along its full length it is making contact with the floor. Continue for a few moments.

- Now tense your body, tightening each part from the tips of your toes to the top of your head as forcefully as you can. Hold this tension for a few moments, then let go, breathing out as you do. You may want to repeat this two or three times.

- On the final repetition, as you breathe out, let go mentally of all your anxieties.

- Feel the weight of your body sinking into the floor and your mind becoming quiet.

- Remain like this for five to ten minutes, or more if you wish.

HYPERTENSION – THE REAL 'KILLER'

You may think that there's nothing to this exercise, and of course you're right. That's the whole point. You are doing nothing; simply resting. But don't make the mistake of thinking that it's doing nothing for you. The corpse posture has proved to be effective in the management of hypertension, or chronically high blood pressure. Raised blood pressure is a normal feature of the stress response. It serves to direct blood more speedily to the brain and limbs so that appropriate action can be taken to deal with a threat or a challenge. Afterwards it quickly returns to normal. This is a healthy and potentially life-saving response. However, if it is repeatedly triggered in response to everyday events, blood pressure remains elevated and over time the condition becomes chronic.

Hypertension is unfortunately very common and potentially deadly, with the long-term effects including cardiovascular disease, which results in heart disease/heart attacks, and temporary or permanent brain damage as a result of stroke. Hypertension also affects the kidneys. The kidneys control blood pressure, but when diseased by hypertension they raise the blood pressure further, establishing a vicious cycle that can result in kidney failure.

THE BENEFITS OF 'CORPSING'

All of these hypertension-induced conditions are potentially fatal. Relaxation is the natural antidote to hypertension. Claims made for the therapeutic and preventative benefits of the corpse posture, tried and tested over many thousand of years in India, have been supported by contemporary medical research. It has proved effective in reducing hypertension even in cases that were unresponsive to drugs. It has been shown to have similar effects to the tranquilliser Diazepam and to be a valid replacement for synthetic drugs that have harmful side-effects. So, next time you feel like having a lie down, just do it.

PILATES

An increasingly popular contemporary approach to exercise based on relaxation is Pilates (pronounced *pi-lah-tis*). This revolutionary approach to exercise and fitness was developed in the 1920s by

Joseph Pilates (1880–1967) who claimed that this method of body conditioning develops the body uniformly, corrects posture, restores vitality, invigorates the mind and elevates the spirit.

The exercises he initially developed were highly specialised, within the capabilities of highly trained dancers and athletes but beyond those of the ordinary person. The exercises prescribed were also tailored to individual needs and for many years remained almost exclusive to all but the wealthy and privileged. However, as the effectiveness of the methods in conditioning the body, preventing skeletal and postural problems and treating stress-related conditions became more widely recognised within orthodox and complementary medicine by physiotherapists, osteopaths and chiropractors, they became much sought after.

During Pilates's lifetime his methods evolved, and continued to do so after his death. His exercises were adapted, simplified and new exercises introduced to make them accessible to a wider and more sedentary clientele. Initial exercises are now simple, comfortable and within anyone's capabilities. They are also slow and controlled.

The Pilates method rebalances the body, altering the way in which muscles are used, restoring natural, normal movement. It also revitalises the body because it reduces the amount of energy lost in keeping muscles tense when not required for an activity. By releasing hidden tension Pilates has a de-stressing effect and, in addition to rebalancing, realigning, replenishing and rejuvenating the body, Pilates also reshapes it, quite dramatically and permanently, improving appearance, self-confidence and self-esteem.

Pilates, in its aims and practices, shares a good deal with traditional yoga. Many of its exercises are almost identical. The major difference is, whereas yoga seems 'foreign', exotic, mystical and mystifying to many people, Pilates is very much a product of its time, and fits neatly with the youth, beauty, health and fitness orientation of contemporary Western culture.

Like yoga, Pilates is a holistic approach, emphasising the need to achieve mastery of the mind in order to gain complete control of the body. It requires constant awareness of how muscles are being used and therefore needs concentration and focus. It is both a mental and physical training method. Relaxation is fundamental to this approach because Joseph Pilates recognised that one of the most important skills you need when exercising is knowing how to work without undue tension. Taking time to relax and release tension from both the mind and the body is the starting point of any Pilates exercise programme. Each Pilates session begins with exercises that heighten the awareness of tensions in the body, especially those normally hidden, and allows them to melt away so that only the muscles needed for specific movements are used.

Exercise 2
Pilates relaxation

Prepare for this exercise as for Exercise 1. You may place a flat firm pillow under your head to allow your neck to maintain its natural curves and prevent its muscles tightening and shortening.

- Lie on your back with your knees bent, hip-width apart and in parallel.

- Place your feet in line with your hips. You may find you are more comfortable when your feet are placed in line with your shoulders.

- Keep your feet parallel and your toes in the same line.
- Open your elbows by placing your hands on your abdomen.
- Soften the balls of the feet and uncurl your toes.
- Soften your ankles.
- Soften the lower part of your legs.
- Release the tension in your thighs.
- Soften the area around your hips.
- Allow your lower back to sink into the floor.
- Feel the length of your spine.
- Stretch your fingers away from your palms and feel the centre of your palms opening before allowing the fingers to curl and the palms soften.
- Let your shoulders widen.
- Soften your breastbone.
- Release your neck.
- Make sure your jaw is loose and free.
- Let your tongue widen at its base and rest comfortably at the bottom of your mouth.
- Ensure that your lips are softly closed.
- Close your eyes.

■ Keep your forehead smooth and free of lines.

■ Soften your face.

■ Allow your whole body to widen and lengthen.

■ Let it sink into the floor.

■ Remain in this position for up to 20 minutes simply allowing all the tension to drain from your body.

When you are ready to get up, gently allow your head to roll to one side. Allow the weight of the head to take it over. Then return your head to the centre and allow it to roll to the other side. Bring it back to the centre once again. Wriggle your fingers and toes, then gently roll on to one side and rest for a few moments before getting up slowly. Bring you head up last.

Ideally, you should aim to practise either of the above relaxation exercises for up to 20 minutes each, twice a day, in order to acquire the habit of releasing tension.

You will find that, with practice, relaxation becomes easier and you will start to feel its benefits. Although you can do either exercise lying down on the floor in front of the television, it is better to use a quiet room or perhaps just some quiet relaxing music in the background. This is because both approaches require concentration and focus in order to identify tension and release it.

Early morning and before going to bed are good times to relax. It might seem strange to recommend relaxing soon after getting out of bed but it is normal for dreaming sleep to occur shortly before waking so the brain is more active and the body less relaxed than in non-dreaming sleep. Relaxing after a warm bath or shower before breakfast can be an ideal way to energise yourself for the day ahead. Similarly, relaxing before going to bed is an excellent way of unwinding and preparing for a good night's sleep. Another good time to relax is when you come in from work and before your evening meal. Making this a habit will enable you to change gear easily from work mode to leisure mode, to leave behind the hassles of the day and re-energise yourself for whatever the evening promises.

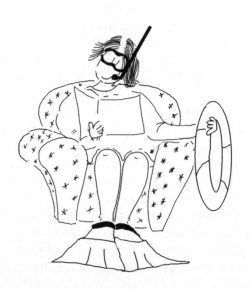

CHAPTER 2

TAKING A BREATHER

Imagine for a moment that you are facing an angry bull across a field and that it begins to run towards you at speed. How would you be breathing? You would almost certainly be taking rapid, shallow breaths. Now imagine that half way towards you the bull is distracted and it stops suddenly, giving you time to leave the field safely. Your first response on reaching safety would be to breathe a sigh of relief, and you would probably take a few really deep breaths as you recover from the ordeal. As you do so your body would gradually relax and you would calm down.

Imagine instead that, having reached safety, you continue to breathe in the same rapid manner as before. If you do this you will remain highly agitated and may even become panicky. When you are stressed, under pressure and tense, you are in a similar state. Although you may not be aware of it, your breathing is rapid and shallow, and confined to your upper chest, which is tense and may feel constricted. Breathing in this way acts as a stressor on your body because it uses only a small amount of available lung capacity and limits the amount of oxygen available to your body cells.

VITAL BREATH

The health of your body depends on the health of its cells. They are the power source that keep the body energised and alive. In addition to its own specialised function, every cell of the body and nervous system produces adenosine triphosphate (ATP), the substance that fuels the body and carries its energy. This process requires oxygen because cells convert it into ATP. Oxygen is therefore the source of all energy in the body. Without it there would be no ATP and without ATP the body would immediately shut down. Constant upper chest breathing reduces the oxygen available for normal cell function and without proper amounts of oxygen ATP is not produced. Consequently, energy is not available to the body.

Chronic shallow chest breathing therefore produces chronic or intermittent fatigue. It is also the first step to disease, because anything that reduces the amount of energy in the body potentially produces disease. Shallow breathing can result in chest pains and palpitations suggestive of heart disease, tingling and numbness in the limbs, muscular cramps in the upper body and back, stomach upsets, heartburn and flatulence, anxiety and panic attacks, feelings of unreality and hallucinations, sleep disturbances, nightmares and night sweats. In fact, shallow breathing compromises the body's metabolism and lowers resistance to disease and can therefore result in virtually any disorder.

If you are someone whose breathing is habitually shallow, you are unlikely to have enough energy or feel well enough to exercise, so, before you can contemplate embarking on exercise, you need to learn how to breathe properly and deliver enough oxygen to your cells to produce the energy they need. With enough energy everything in life becomes possible, including exercise. All traditional and contemporary approaches to health and fitness recognise that overall health relies on breathing efficiency.

AEROBIC EXERCISE

Aerobic exercise, which literally means 'with oxygen', gives your body more oxygen for energy. It also conditions the body, promotes endurance, burns fat, thereby assisting weight loss, and increases the metabolic rate so that the body uses fat as its primary fuel. However, most people breathe incorrectly, using only a fraction of their lung capacity, and have to be taught how to breathe properly.

BREATHING TECHNIQUES

In the East, breathing techniques are fundamental to traditional healthcare systems that emphasise preventative medicine and self-help. Hatha yoga promotes the optimal flow and balance of energy through various postures and flowing movements, and breathing exercises called *pranayama*. In China, *T'ai Chi Chuan* is a gentle system of physical and breathing exercises, widely practised, as is *Qi Gong* which focuses on removing energy blockages. The Japanese equivalents, *Do-In* and *Ge Jo*, combine breathing techniques with physical massage and stretching. All these practices are both relaxing and highly energising and breathing techniques are a key component of Chinese and Japanese martial arts which are physically demanding, involving considerable exertion and explosive but controlled movements.

The method of breathing emphasised in these approaches is from the belly rather than the chest. As the breath goes in, the belly starts rising, and as the breath goes out, the belly settles down. This is how babies breathe and how we breathe when asleep, but not how most of us breathe when awake. *'When the belly rises up, it is really the life energy, the spring of life that is rising and falling down with each breath'* (C. Gosselin, *The Ultimate Guide to Fitness*).

The richest blood flow is in the lower lungs and if air does not reach this area the body's cells do not receive enough oxygen. Proper breathing requires the full use of the diaphragm, the layer of muscle that separates the chest and abdominal cavities. When you breathe correctly the diaphragm contracts and the abdomen expands, allowing the lungs to fill with air. Breathing from the diaphragm also stimulates and assists the body's waste mechanism, the lymph system. A deep diaphragmic breath therefore both energises and cleanses the entire system. Modern scientific understanding confirms the ancient belief that belly breathing is best, and contemporary approaches to health emphasise the importance of learning to breathe deeply in this way.

The following exercises are based on both traditional and contemporary practices.

Exercise 3
Belly breathing

This exercise is a feature of traditional Indian *Vipassana* practice, a means of promoting the awareness of the essence of life or being. It is very simple and yet highly effective in relaxing the mind and the body while energising both.

- Lie or sit comfortably with head and body aligned and straight.

- Close your eyes and breathe normally.

- Stay as still as possible, changing position only if really necessary.

■ Having done this, simply observe the rise and fall of your belly slightly above the navel as you breathe in and out.

■ Don't worry about distractions; thoughts, feelings and body sensations will arise. Simply note them and return to watching your belly rising and falling.

■ Continue to observe your breathing in this way for 20 minutes.

An alternative method is to focus attention on the tip of your nose and observe as you breathe in and out of your nostrils.

Exercise 4
The breathing corpse

This exercise combines basic breathing techniques with the *savasana* posture (see Chapter 1).

■ Lie on the floor with your head and body aligned, legs parallel and feet together.

■ Allow your legs and feet to roll away from each other.

■ Stretch your arms alongside the body but not touching it, hands palm up and fingers curled slightly inwards.

■ Close your eyes and let go mentally.

■ Remain this way for around five minutes, allowing your body to sink into the floor and your mind to become quiet.

■ Allow your eyeballs to sink back into their sockets.

■ Smooth any wrinkles in your forehead and face.

■ Relax your jaw, opening your mouth slightly and keeping your teeth slightly apart.

- Rest your tongue on the lower palate and keep it still. As it relaxes, allow the base of your tongue to recede into your throat.

- Allow the tightness in your neck to dissolve.

- Press your shoulders down and move the shoulder blades into the back ribs. As you do so, lower your chin slightly towards your throat, lengthening the back of your neck.

- When your body feels relaxed, focus on your breathing. Observe it in your chest. Be aware of its rhythm. Notice whether your breathing is deep or shallow, fast or slow, regular or irregular, soft or harsh, noisy or quiet. Are your inhalations and exhalations the same length?

- Remain lying quietly, simply observing as you gently breathe in and out.

- Avoid any tendency to become tense as you breathe. If you move your head backwards as you breathe in, or tighten your abdomen, hands or feet as you breathe out, release this tension with each out-breath.

You are now ready to deepen your relaxation. To do so:

- Breathe out and relax your abdomen.

- Exhale slowly and quietly without straining.

- Continue breathing in and out slowly and quietly for about five minutes.

- Now, breathe out completely and take a slow, quiet in-breath. Don't breathe in sharply or deeply. Breathe out normally.

- Now breathe in slowly and quietly. Make this a long in-breath and make sure that you don't tense your eyes or flare your nostrils as you do so.

- Breathe out normally. Continue breathing like this for five minutes.

- When you have done this, breathe out completely, emptying your lungs.

- Breathe in slowly and quietly, lengthening the breath gradually. Then exhale slowly and fully. Continue to breathe in this rhythm for five minutes without tightening any part of your face and body.

- Now breathe normally, before slowly rolling on to your side with knees bent before standing up.

Exercise 5
Pilates thoracic breathing

If asked to take a deep breath most people lift their chest high, raise their shoulders and arch their upper back. This uses only the upper part of the lungs and doesn't fully oxygenate the cells of the body and enable them to function optimally. Pilates teaches a thoracic breathing technique, so called because it uses the chest and back muscles to expand the chest and ribs fully, that greatly improves breathing effectiveness.

You can try this sitting, standing or lying down.

- Wrap a towel around your ribs, crossing it over in front.

- Holding each end of the towel, pull it gently tight and breathe in allowing your ribs to expand the towel. Avoid lifting the breastbone too high.

- As you breathe out, gently squeeze the towel to help you empty your lungs and relax your rib cage.

When you have mastered this breathing technique you can dispense with the towel:

- Lie down in the relaxation position (see Chapter 1), with head and body aligned, knees bent, legs parallel, toes in a line, arms bent at the side of the body, and hands resting palm down on the lower abdomen.

- While breathing as described above, allow your entire body to sink into the floor.

- As you breathe out, allow your body to widen and lengthen.

- Breathe in and, as you breathe out, soften the feet, uncurling your toes and ankles.

- With each out-breath, progressively release the tightness in your lower legs, knees, thighs and hips, feeling the body lengthen along the spine as you do so.

- Ensure that your lower back sinks into the floor.

- On an out-breath allow the shoulder blades to widen and the front of your shoulders to soften.

- Let your breastbone soften also.

- Breathe out and widen your elbows, and with successive out-breaths, stretch your fingers away from your palms and feel them opening.

- Release your neck and jaw.

- Let your tongue widen at its base and rest comfortably at the bottom of your mouth.

- Close your eyes and allow your face to become soft and smooth.

- Simply observe your breathing, ensuring that you continue to breathe widely and fully, releasing any residual tension from your muscles as breathe out.

- Continue to do so for 10–20 minutes.

- When you have done so, roll on to one side with knees bent and get up slowly.

Exercise 6
Power breathing

Power breathing can be used to increase energy at any time. It can also be used to reduce tension, pain and anxiety. You can perform this exercise lying, sitting or standing.

- Place one of your hands a little above your waist.

- Breathe in slowly to the count of one, allowing your diaphragm to expand and your lungs to fill with air. As they do so, your hand should move upwards (if you are lying down) or forwards if you are sitting or standing.

- When the diaphragm has expanded to its full extent, hold your breath to the count of four, then slowly exhale to the count of two, allowing your diaphragm and hand to return to the resting position.

■ Repeat 10 times.

As you become familiar with this technique, you can increase the count for each stage of the exercise but keep the ratio the same – 1:4:2; for example, breathe in to the count of *5*, hold breath to the count of *20* and breathe out to the count of *10*. Ideally, to boost energy you should take 10 power breaths three times daily.

Deep breathing is often recommended as a way of reducing tension, pain and anxiety. Tension tightens and narrows the chest and throat, resulting in shallow breathing. In principle therefore, attempting to breathe deeply should reverse the process, as it requires a relaxation of tension in these areas. In practice, however, it often has quite the opposite effect. Uncertainty about where to focus when attending to breathing can generate anxiety and increase tension, as can the strangeness of deep breathing if your breathing is habitually shallow. As a result, tension can tighten your chest further and induce a sense of panic. While such a reaction is not uncommon, more typically, people find that their attention is diverted from their breathing by intrusive thoughts and they may become anxious because of their inability to focus. Worrying about being unable to relax makes them more tense.

If you encounter any of these problems when attempting breathing techniques you may benefit from relaxation methods that encourage deep breathing while distracting your attention from breathing itself. The exercises in the next chapter employ sound to this effect.

CHAPTER 3

SOUNDS RELAXING

Have you ever tried to walk out of step with a military band? If you haven't, try it. It's virtually impossible. Whether or not you are aware of it, all music has mental and physical effects because your natural biological rhythms synchronise with it. Music is a natural pacemaker. You 'hear' it throughout your body because the auditory nerve connects the inner ear with all the muscles of the body. So muscle strength, flexibility and tone are influenced by sound and vibration. Music in the lower frequencies resonates in the lower back region, pelvis, thighs and legs, and as the frequencies increase you feel them more in the upper chest, neck and head.

Heart rate responds to frequency, tempo and volume and tends to speed up or slow down to match the rhythm of a sound. Athletes often choose music with a tempo to match their target heart rate. If they are aiming to achieve a heart rate of 170 beats per minute in training they will listen to music with that rhythm. Softer music with a slower tempo reduces the heartbeat and is calming. Music with a strong beat can raise body temperature by a few degrees, while soft music with a weak beat can lower it. So music can literally help you warm up *and* cool down.

Music also affects respiration. Breathing rate is normally 25–35 breaths a minute but it increases in response to fast loud music. This is achieved by shallower breathing. As fast, shallow breathing is a feature of stress and anxiety, it is associated with increased mental and physical tension and can produce scattered thinking, impulsive behaviour, a tendency to make mistakes, and accident proneness and, as explained in the previous chapter, shallow breathing can also result in the cells of the body receiving insufficient oxygen.

A deeper, slower rate of breathing contributes to calmness, greater emotional and physical control and improved energy metabolism. By listening to music with a slower tempo or with longer, slower sounds, you can slow and deepen breathing. This not only calms the body and mind but also oxygenates the cells of the body, producing energy and boosting the immune system.

Music can also slow down brain wave activity – the slower the brain waves, the more relaxed, peaceful and contented you feel – and can increase the level of endorphins, chemicals produced naturally by the body that reduce feelings of anxiety and pain, and produce a natural 'high'. It can also regulate stress hormones.

MAKING YOUR OWN MUSIC

Rhythmic auditory stimuli such as drumming, singing, humming, chanting and intoning – making elongated vowel sounds – have been widely employed in rituals in most cultures throughout history to generate changes in brain wave patterns and alter states of awareness. Buddhist monks and Tibetan yogis have a long tradition of chanting or intoning certain sounds to induce altered mental and physical states, typically using short phrases or words. Some, like the Hindu *om*, which comprises the three basic sounds A-U-M from which all sounds are derived, is considered to produce the same effect for anyone who intones it correctly, but it is also recognised that individuals vary with regard to which particular sounds are most helpful to them.

Some of the effects attributed to chanting, intoning and humming can be understood in terms of the resonance between the vibrational patterns created and the natural rhythms of the body. They calm the mind and stabilise brain and body rhythms. However, many of the beneficial effects attributed to these practices are a consequence of increased oxygenation of the body resulting from the improved breathing patterns they encourage.

SOUND EXERCISES

The exercises in this chapter all use self-generated sound as an aid to relaxation. It is better to sit rather than lie down for these exercises. Find somewhere where you will not be disturbed. Sit down and take a few moments to become aware of how you feel. Are you comfortable? Do you feel impatient, or anxious? As you identify your feelings adjust your position so you sit as comfortably as you can.

Now, close your eyes. Bring your attention to your body boundaries, to the contact your body makes with surrounding surfaces – your clothes, your shoes, the chair, cushions or floor. You will probably find that you are not as comfortable as you first supposed. Your clothes or shoes may feel restrictive. If so, loosen tight garments, remove shoes, and spectacles if you are wearing them.

Notice also your posture. Most people, when they sit 'comfortably', impose a great deal of unnecessary tension and strain on their bodies, principally by sitting without adequate support for the back. If you are sitting on a chair or against a wall you may find that you are leaning against the back of the chair or wall and your lower back has minimal contact with it. Adjust your position so that your back, trunk and legs are well supported. Ideally, the seat of a chair should be the same length as your thighs and your lower back should be tucked into the angle of the chair. Ensure that there is no large gap between your lower back and supporting surfaces, and that your back is straight.

Lengthen your neck so that your head is upright and your chin isn't pulled down towards your chest.

Probably your hands, arms, legs or ankles are folded or crossed. This involves muscle tension, so reduce this by uncrossing your limbs. If sitting on a chair, place your feet apart and firmly on the ground, rest your arms on your thighs or the arms of the chair so that no parts of the body are twisted or crossed. If sitting on the floor extend your legs in front of you, feet apart, and allow your feet to fall to the side. Rest your arms and hands on your thighs.

When you have made yourself comfortable, close your eyes, or, if you prefer to keep your eyes open, sit facing a plain wall about an arm's length away. Gaze softly at the wall. Sitting in this way will help you to relax and to produce sound freely. Keeping your eyes closed or focused on a plain wall helps to avoid distractions and to maintain focus on the exercise you are attempting.

Exercise 7
Humming

Nadabrahma is an ancient Tibetan technique that was originally performed for an hour very early every morning. However, it can be practised at any time of the day and as little as five minutes can help you relax.

■ Start humming out loud and create a vibration throughout your body. You can change the pitch of the humming and move your body smoothly and slowly if you feel like it. You may simply wish to continue humming in this way for 10–20 minutes.

Traditionally, the exercise has three further stages:

Stage 1: Here, the idea is that you are releasing into the universe the energy held in as tension. It may help to think of this as you perform the movements.

■ After several minutes humming, move your hands palm upwards in an outward circular motion, starting at the navel.

■ Move both hands forward together and then part them to make two large circles mirroring each other left and right. The movement should be so slow as to be almost imperceptible.

■ Continue to do this for five minutes

Stage 2: During these movements think that you are taking energy in from the universe and becoming more and more energised.

■ Turn your hands palms down and start moving them in the opposite direction so that your hands come together at the navel and part outwards to the sides of the body. As in the first stage, don't inhibit any soft, slow movements of the rest of your body.

■ Continue for five minutes.

Stage 3:

■ Sit absolutely quiet and still for a few minutes.

You can continue with each stage for as long as you wish, or you can spend five minutes on each.

Exercise 8
Intoning

■ Sit comfortably with your eyes closed.

■ Allow yourself to relax and when you feel ready, intone loudly and outwardly the three sounds *Aaaa – Uuuu – Mmmm* combining them into one continuous sound.

■ As you repeat the sounds, elongate each of them (*Aaaaaaa – Uuuuuuu – Mmmmmmm*). You will find that they combine to make the sound *oh-um*.

■ Allow yourself to attune with the sound and to be filled by it. Forget everything else.

■ As you repeat it, become the sound. Allow it to vibrate through your body and mind, and through your entire nervous system. Intone it and feel as if every cell of your body is vibrating with it.

When you begin to feel harmonious with the sound, you can stop intoning loudly. Close your lips and intone the sounds inwardly. Intone inwardly but loudly so that the sound spreads through your body. Allow yourself to feel vitalised by the sound, as if you are an instrument.

As you feel the sounds more intensely, begin to slow them down and make them more subtle and soft. Continue to intone the sounds in this way until you feel deeply relaxed.

Exercise 9
Going do-lally

Many relaxation exercises focus on relaxing the body, but they meet with only limited success if the mind is not also relaxed. This is because the contents of mind – recurrent thoughts and worries, anxieties, concerns and preoccupations – give rise to physical tensions. True relaxation can therefore only be attained if you can let go of these mental activities.

Traditionally this has been achieved by repeating syllables or sounds that have no intrinsic meaning. This occupies the mind with a content-free subject and enables the body to relax and release the energy held in tension. Any syllables or sounds can be used. *Devavani* is a traditional practice that makes use of the sound *la*.

- Sit quietly with eyes closed for up to five minutes. You may wish to have gentle music playing in the background.

- Begin to repeat the sounds 'la la la' and continue for up to five minutes.

- Allow your body to move in harmony with the sounds. Other nonsense sounds may be produced quite spontaneously. Continue for up to five minutes.

- Lie down and remain silent and still for five minutes.

Exercise 10
Having a good laugh

Though laughter has long been considered the best medicine, claims about the beneficial effects of laughter have only been investigated in recent years. It is now established that laughter does have measurable physical effects. It reduces the hormones cortisol and adrenaline, whose levels increase in response to stress, and also stimulates the release of endorphins, the neurotransmitters that stimulate the pleasure centre in the brain, promoting feelings of well-being and relaxation.

A 'good' laugh also exercises the muscles of the face, shoulders, diaphragm and abdomen, and more robust laughter involves the arm and leg muscles. It has been claimed that laughing 100–200 times a day is equal to about 10 minutes of rowing. 'Hearty' laughter speeds up heart rate, raises blood pressure, accelerates breathing and oxygen consumption. It produces similar 'huffing and puffing' to exercise, and has been described as 'internal jogging'. As laughter subsides it is followed by a brief period of relaxation during which respiration and heart rate slow down, often to below normal levels, blood pressure drops and muscles relax.

The most vigorous kind of laughter involves the belly. Few people today allow themselves a real 'belly laugh' because of the associated physical reactions of heaving stomach and sides, streaming eyes, doubled-up posture and falling about.

A traditional Hindu exercise produces similar effects to belly laughter. It simply requires you to focus on breathing at your stomach and to repeat the syllable *Ha* on each out-breath. Very quickly this leads to a 'belly' laugh and produces relaxation.

A variation of this exercise is to sit or lie down, close your eyes and bring your attention to your stomach. Imagine that you have a large red clown's nose held there by a piece of elastic and that as you breathe in and out you can see it move backwards and forwards if you are sitting, or up and down if you are lying down. Breathe in and out deeply for a few minutes watching in your mind the movements of the red nose and noting your reactions. Then on each out-breath repeat the syllable *Ha*. Allow yourself to relax into the rhythm of this repeated sound and as you do so you will begin to laugh. Allow yourself to surrender to the laughter for as long as you can.

If you find that you can't laugh despite attempting this exercise several times, it could well be that you normally repress laughter through tension in your belly region and need to learn to relax more.

Exercise 11
The relaxation response

The traditional use of sound as an aid to relaxation has been adapted into a simple and effective technique by Herbert Benson, an American Professor of Medicine. Professor Benson insists that the ability to relax is an inborn human capacity rather than a skill that requires learning. He calls his method 'the relaxation response'. It has been widely used within medicine in treating a wide range of conditions related to stress and tension.

To elicit the relaxation response:

- Sit comfortably in a quiet environment.

- Close your eyes or focus your attention in a fixed point or object.

- Become aware of your breathing by inhaling through your nose and exhaling through your mouth.

- On each out-breath silently repeat the word 'one'.

- Repeat this pattern up to 20 minutes. During this time don't 'try' to relax, or worry about achieving relaxation. Simply maintain a passive mental attitude. Don't dwell on distracting thoughts or sensations. Acknowledge them if they occur but return your attention to breathing and repeating 'one'.

If, after tr.ying the above exercises, you still find it difficult to relax, you may have residual tension within your body. Apart from preventing relaxation, this tension will continue to drain your energy. Even if you have achieved some degree of relaxation through any of the exercises recommended so far, you will probably retain some tension in your muscles, without even being aware of it. To become aware of this residual or baseline tension and release it, you need to focus attention on your muscles and develop muscle sense. Learn how by trying the exercises in Chapter 4.

CHAPTER 4

TAKING IT EASY

If you have tried the exercises so far you may feel you have now achieved greater calm and feel more energised. But if you haven't been able to relax successfully using these methods, don't despair. This is by no means unusual. True relaxation is not a 'normal' state; it doesn't occur spontaneously but must be consciously and purposely evoked. It is a complex integrated combination of changes in skin resistance, brain wave and breathing patterns, reduced muscle activity, heart and pulse rate, blood pressure and blood hormone levels, and is therefore not a common experience.

PROGRESSIVE RELAXATION

The physician Edmund Jacobsen first systematically investigated relaxation during the 1920s. He established that relaxation is a *progressive* elimination of muscle tension, a process that takes time.

To relax, you need to know not only that you *are* tense but also where exactly the tension is located, how tense you are, and how you are producing and maintaining the tension. Dr Jacobsen devised 'progressive relaxation' to develop bodily awareness, or muscle sense, in individuals to help them relax by becoming more observant of the muscle tension in their bodies, progressively relieving it by a technique of tensing and then releasing the muscles.

Dr Jacobsen used the technique successfully in the treatment of many medical conditions such as hypertension, insomnia, anxiety, and heart disease and recommended it as particularly suitable for cases of fatigue, exhaustion, debility and sleep disturbances.

Some people are not successful in cultivating muscle sense and fail to gain control, usually because they don't practise enough. Indeed, there are some factors that make progressive relaxation unattractive or unsuitable for some individuals, and these are examined at the end of this chapter. If you try progressive relaxation but don't find it particularly successful, consider these factors and then see if you have more success with the approach to relaxation in Chapter 5.

Exercise 12
Letting go of tension

This exercise may seem very lengthy but it can easily be achieved within 20 minutes. Initially, you may find it helpful to have someone read the instructions slowly to you or you could record the instructions and listen to them when you attempt the exercise.

■ Find somewhere you can sit or lie with a reasonable degree of comfort: not so comfortable you drift off to sleep, but not so uncomfortable or cold that you can't sustain the motivation to achieve relaxation.

■ Close your eyes or, if this is difficult because of contact lenses, focus on a fixed point within your line of vision, such as a mark on a wall or floor.

■ Gradually draw your attention from your surroundings and bring it to the boundary between your body and adjacent surfaces. Notice whether the contact is uncomfortable or painful and adjust your position to maximise comfort and minimise pain. You may find that you need to remove restrictive clothing, shoes, jewellery and spectacles. At any point during the exercise, when you feel the need to adjust your position to reduce discomfort or pain, do so.

■ Turn your attention to your feelings. How do you feel? Do you feel silly, or guilty about taking time to do the exercise? How self-conscious are you? Are you worried about being seen by others, about falling asleep, or that you may not be able to 'do' the exercise? Are you already telling yourself you won't achieve relaxation? Your reactions may reflect some of the basic anxieties in your life resulting in some of the tensions you identify as you proceed with the exercise. If, during any part of the exercise, thoughts, feelings, memories or impressions come to mind, make a mental note of them as they may have similar significance.

■ Bring your attention to your toes. Without moving the overall position of your feet, push your toes down and away from you as far as they will go, noticing as you do so the effect of this movement on the rest of your feet and legs. Sustain this tension until you can identify the extent of its effects throughout your body, and then let go of it. Repeat this contraction three times, or as many times as is necessary for you to become aware of its full implications for the rest of your body.

■ Now flex your toes upwards and towards you as far as you can, and sustain this tension until you can feel its effects, not only locally in your feet and legs, but also in more distant areas of your body. Then simply let go of it. Repeat three times.

■ Now rotate each foot in a full circle, first in one direction, then the other, noting any accompanying sensations. Then stop this movement, and for a few moments simply experience the sensations in your feet and legs.

It is important to recognise the sensation of 'letting go' in contrast to that of tightening or tensing, and how both are achieved. The contractions are sustained in order to increase your awareness of how muscle tension is achieved in any given muscle group and the effects it has on other parts of the body. This may highlight habitual tensions and pain, and make you more aware of the situations in which these pains occur. The contractions therefore have implications for the mind/body system as a whole.

■ Turn your attention to your knees. Tighten them and hold that contraction, noticing what parts of your body are involved in this tension. Then let go of it. Repeat three times.

■ Bring your attention to your thighs. Press them firmly downwards against the chair or floor, noting the extent of this action throughout your body. When you have identified the furthest point of influence, let go of the tension. Repeat three times.

■ Without moving the overall position of your legs, draw your inner thighs together and hold them thus, once again noticing the effects of this tension on the rest of your body before letting it go. Repeat three times.

- Bring your attention to your buttocks and press down as hard as you can. Then let go. Repeat three times, noting the effects on your body.

- Draw in or dimple the sides of the buttocks and sustain this contraction until you are aware of its implications for the remainder of your body, then let it go. Repeat three times.

- Allow your legs and feet to flop and take a few seconds to become aware of the sensations within them. If you discover any residual tension work to release it by tightening the relevant muscles then letting go of them. Allow the resulting floppy feeling to spread throughout your lower limbs.

- Take your attention to your lower back. Without shifting your overall position, push it against the adjacent surface and hold it there. It is particularly important to notice the effect this movement has on the rest of your body because the lower back is a major stress point where bodily tensions and pain are often felt. When you have done so, let go and repeat three times.

- Push your lower back forward as far as you can, arching it and holding this tension until you can feel its effects throughout your body. Repeat the action three times.

- Alternate the two movements, and repeat several times before letting go.

- Bring your attention to your navel. Pull it in towards your backbone and hold it until you can feel the effect on your body. Repeat three times slowly and then several times quite quickly as if you are belly dancing. Continue until this movement is becoming slightly unpleasant, then let yourself flop and allow this sensation to spread through your body.

- Take your attention to your chest and observe your breathing and its effects on your body.

- Breathe in deeply and slowly before breathing out slowly.

- Take your attention to your shoulders. Raise them to your ears and hold them in that position. Then drop them. Repeat three times.

- Raise each shoulder independently. Rotate each shoulder through a full circle and then both shoulders together, observing the effect.

- Bring your attention down your right arm to your hand. Make your hand into a fist and tighten it as firmly as you can. Follow this tension as it progresses through your hand, lower arm, upper arm, shoulder, neck, head, jaw and chest. Further tighten your fist so that you can feel its effects in your legs. When you have done this, uncurl your right hand.

- Clasp your left hand and tighten both hands together in a firm grip and notice the effect on your hands, arms, shoulders, neck, head and upper body. Then drop your right hand.

- Form a fist with your left hand. Clench it as tightly as you can, following the tension as it spreads through your arm, shoulder, neck, head and body. Tighten the fist so you can feel its effects in your legs. Then uncurl your fingers and let your hands fall to your sides. Now, press down with your hands as forcefully as you can, noticing the effect on your body. Sustain this tension for several seconds, then let your hands flop. Allow this sensation to spread through your body.

- Take your attention to your neck. Shift your head to the right and hold this position for a few seconds before shifting it to the left.

- Slowly rotate your head through a full circle. Be aware of the effort involved in keeping your head upright before allowing your head to flop forward.

- Bring your attention up your neck and across your scalp. Try and wiggle your scalp and ears if you can.

- Raise your eyebrows and keep them raised as you notice the effect on the rest of your head and face.

- Drop your brows and pull them down towards your chin, and hold them there. Feel the effects on your head and neck before letting go.

- Bringing your attention to your nose, flare your nostrils as widely as possible.

- Tighten your nostrils.

- Press your lips tightly together noticing the effects on your face.

- Clench your teeth as tightly as possible. Notice the effects of this action on the muscles of your face, head, neck and chest.

- Shift your jaw from side to side. Notice the effects on the temples. Let your mouth hang open. Breathe in through your nose and out through your open mouth. Continue to breathe like this for a few moments.

- Bring your attention back to your feet. Scan your body upwards noting any tightness, discomfort or pain in any region and release the tension by alternately tightening and letting go of it. If the tightness or discomfort persists make a mental note because this needs to be dealt with before full relaxation can be achieved.

- To the count of *1* let go of the tightness in your feet and legs; *2* let go of the tightness in your lower back and abdomen; *3* let go of the tightness in your shoulders, arms, hands and chest; *4* let go of your head; and *5* let go of the tightness in your jaw.

- Spend a minute or so becoming aware of the sensations throughout your body. If relaxed your body should feel heavy and warm. Allow yourself to enjoy this feeling for as long as you wish.

The exercise above is a very effective way of letting go of tension in your muscles. If, having tried it, you still haven't been able to relax, you might not be putting enough effort into tightening your muscles. But sometimes the problem is not lack of effort. It may be that your muscles are habitually so tense that you can't make them any tighter than they already are. The existing tension in a muscle group may be such that any attempt to tighten that area produces pain. However, this can also produce insights. Sometimes the discovery of so much existing tension in certain areas of the body can enable you to release tension there. Tension is a way that the body protects itself from pain and injury and releasing tension can make you aware of pain or injury that has been masked by it.

If the exercise above seems to lengthy for you, try this shorter but still effective way of releasing tension. It can be done when lying in bed at night before sleep or when watching television.

Exercise 13
Loosening up

■ Position yourself as comfortably as possible and focus your attention on your toes. Tighten them for a few seconds and then loosen them. Repeat this once or twice.

■ Move your attention to your lower legs, tighten the muscles there and hold that tightness for a few seconds before loosening it.

■ Work your way upwards, tightening and loosening each of the major areas of your body in turn: your thighs, buttocks, lower back, stomach, chest, shoulders, arms, hands, neck, face and jaw.

■ If any parts of your body remain tense, tight or painful, spend a few minutes alternately tightening and loosening them until you feel an overall reduction of tightness in your body.

■ Once again focus attention on your toes. Tighten them, and while still doing so proceed to tighten your calves, thighs, buttocks, lower back, stomach, chest, shoulders, arms, hands, neck, face and jaw so that your muscles become progressively tighter from the tip of your toes to the point of your jaw.

- Continue to tighten your muscles until your body has become quite rigid. Hold this stiffness for a few moments and then let go of it.

- Take a few moments to experience the sensation throughout your body. If you have been really tightening your muscles your body should be quite floppy once you let go.

- Repeat this exercise twice more. Each time try to tighten your muscles more than on the previous occasion. After the third repetition, provided you have really worked at tightening your muscles, your body should feel pleasantly relaxed and loosened up. Allow yourself to enjoy the experience for as long as you wish, noting any parts of the body where tension tends to creep back. Make a mental note of these areas because they are likely to be the 'stress' points where tension habitually occurs, and the major drain on your energy.

RELAXATION NOT PROGRESSING?

Although relaxation procedures that focus on muscle tensing can be highly effective, many people find the approach not necessarily painful but definitely painfully boring. If you have tried relaxing in this way and found yourself becoming impatient or bored, and more tense as a result, it might be worthwhile pausing to consider what you are so impatient about that it prevents you relaxing. Remember: relaxation is the opposite of doing. It is non-doing, or even more precisely undoing – it involves undoing the muscular tension in the body, like *undoing* knots in a piece of string by working them loose. It takes time, and if you don't make or take time for relaxation, you will not achieve it.

You may be impatient to get on and do other things that you feel you *should* be doing. If so, ask yourself what these things are, whether you actually *need* to do them right now and why you feel you must. In other words, begin by relaxing your attitude to doing: focus on it and work on it, just like working on relaxing your body. Although the mind is not a muscle, as some people claim, it does work in the same way in that it tends towards certain habitual, learned patterns. These ways of thinking become 'second nature', and set up patterns of behaviour that are quite unnecessary and often unhelpful. By focusing attention on the *shoulds* and *should nots* of your life, you may be able to let go of many of them and adopt a more relaxed outlook and approach to living.

A further drawback of relaxation procedures that focus on muscle tightening is that they can create greater tension and anxiety. Most people find it easier to tighten their muscles than to loosen them because this is habitual behaviour. So when they increase the tension in their bodies they tend to retain it. This is particularly true of those people who most need to learn how to relax. Their overall level of tension is therefore increased rather than reduced and this produces anxiety, panic or other unpleasant feelings.

If you are being affected this way, you may be unable to relax using procedures – like progressive relaxation – that focus primarily on muscle tension. Even if you can achieve relaxation this way to some extent, you may still experience sudden anxiety and even panic. This is because the effects associated with relaxation, which can include sensations of wooziness, lightness, falling, floating, vibrations, tingling or loss of feeling in limbs, will appear strange if you have rarely or never experienced them before.

You may have found that emphasis on the muscle groups of the body interferes with relaxation because you keep thinking about them. This can be counterproductive because one of the main aims of any approach to relaxation is to reduce thinking, which is simply another 'doing'.

It may just be that the physicality of progressive relaxation is not suited to you. You might benefit from a quite different approach, as presented in Chapter 5.

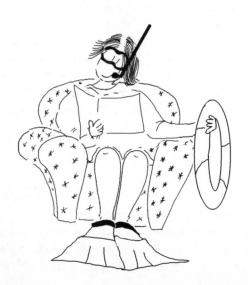

CHAPTER 5

LETTING YOUR MIND WANDER

VISUALISATION

With the exception of a tiny minority of people with certain kinds of brain damage, everyone relies heavily on the ability to think in pictures. We all base choices and decisions on our ability to form mental pictures or visual images, and this is known as visualisation. Without it, everyday life as we know it would be impossible. We decide what clothes to wear by picturing how we will look in them, we picture how fixtures and fittings will look in our home, we imagine our holiday before we've even chosen a destination. The ability to think in visual images also enables us to picture our self, our past, present and future. It determines self-identity and self-image.

Thinking in pictures provides us with an important tool for acquiring and processing knowledge. Visualisation gives us, quite literally, a different way of looking at our self and the world, and when combined with verbal reasoning, it increases the flexibility of our mental processes and greatly enhances our intellectual capabilities. The ability to 'see' the nature of reality and solutions to problems in this way appears to be the key to all creative ability.

The brain is unable to distinguish between seeing in the mind's eye and seeing in the external world. The brain and the body therefore respond in the same way to visual images as they do to visual perception. Images have direct physiological effects. We salivate when we imagine eating a lemon, and sexual and fearful images produce dramatic physiological reactions. Visual images can produce changes in blood flow, blood sugar levels, blood pressure, levels of blood hormones and cholesterol, heart rate, gastrointestinal activity, perspiration, muscle tension, breathing, eye movements, pupil size, and can affect the functioning of the immune system. Visual images also affect the musculo-skeletal system; for instance, imagining lifting progressively heavy weights produces an increase in muscle tension.

It is therefore possible to induce physiological effects by way of the imagination. Doing this deliberately to bring about physiological changes by way of the psychological and physical and emotional information conveyed by visual images is known as active or creative imagination. One way in which this can be used to bring about physiological change is by inducing relaxation. It can do this because it is highly absorbing and any activity that engages and occupies our attention is also relaxing. The manner in which visual images form instantaneously and simultaneously in the mind results in a time sense quite unrelated to clock time. This relieves stress and pressure associated with time, and because it also helps reduce reliance on ordinary verbal thinking, visualisation also relieves the physical tensions that arise from mental anxieties.

Visualisation is now used as an effective aid to physical achievement and fitness. Creating an image of something you want to achieve provides a stimulus that gives you a clear and positive goal and focusing on this image in your mind's eye regularly and consistently can help you overcome fears and other obstacles to that goal. Positive mental images encourage positive behaviour. In spite of having read this far, you might still be holding on to the negative belief that exercise is difficult and not enjoyable: it will never work for you so there's no point in trying. Now, for a change, just try imagining yourself enjoying exercising and imagine seeing great results afterwards. If you adopt a positive outlook you are much more likely to exercise and improve your fitness. And you won't have to consider yourself lazy any more – after all, isn't that why you're here?

Practise the following exercises, which use your imagination as an aid to breathing, relaxation and motivation.

Exercise 14
Breathing lightly

By itself, breathing through the nose slows and deepens breathing and produces greater relaxation. Nevertheless for many people, initially at least, it may not be sufficiently absorbing to hold their attention. Imagining breathing in light or colour is much more absorbing for most people and produces relaxation more easily.

- Find somewhere to sit or lie comfortably and close your eyes or focus on a fixed point within your line of vision – a mark on the ceiling, wall or floor.

- Gradually draw your attention from your surroundings and bring it to the boundary between your body and the adjacent surfaces. As you do so, notice whether the contact is uncomfortable and adjust your position to maximise comfort.

- When you are positioned as comfortably as possible, focus attention on the tip of your nose. Imagine that you are breathing coloured light in through your nose. It enters your body and is drawn in and through your head and from your head along the length of the spine to its base, where it curls upwards.

■ As you breathe out, the coloured light is drawn upwards, forcing all your tension in the form of a dark dense fog towards and out of your mouth, leaving your body full of coloured light and feeling relaxed, light and clear.

■ Continue breathing in this way until you feel fully relaxed and at ease.

If during this exercise you find that there are parts of your head and body where the imaginary light seems blocked or through which it can't pass easily, it is likely that these are areas of tension. Focusing attention on these areas so that the imaginary light can pass will help to relieve the tension. You may then identify areas of tension that you are usually unaware of. Relaxing them in this way helps to alleviate tension headaches and other painful conditions associated with muscle tension.

Exercise 15
Dissolving tension

■ Find somewhere you can sit or lie comfortably and close your eyes or focus on a fixed point.

■ Imagine you are outdoors on a warm sunny day. The heat from the sun is pleasant and you can feel its rays gently warming your body.

■ As you become aware of your body and sensations within it, identify areas of tension, discomfort or pain. Imagine these in the form of ice.

- As you focus your attention on each of these areas in turn, imagine that the sun's rays are penetrating your body and melting the ice. Your tensions, discomforts or pains dissolve, first into drops and then a trickle, and eventually into a stream of fluid that flows through and out of your body, leaving it feeling pleasantly warm and heavy.

- When your bodily tensions have disappeared, focus on your head. Imagine that the sun's rays are penetrating your mind and dissolving your mental tensions and anxieties. They too flow away through and out of your body, leaving your mind clear.

- Allow yourself a few minutes to observe and experience the flow within you.

- Imagine that the sun's rays penetrating your head are now dissolving all the obstacles in your mind to undertaking exercising, improving your level of fitness and becoming more healthy.

- As these mental blockages to exercise disappear, allow yourself to feel that you want to exercise.

- Imagine exercising in a way that feels easy and enjoyable.

- Imagine yourself becoming fitter and more energetic.

- Imagine how the new fitter you feels and looks. Hold this image in your mind. Allow it to become bigger and brighter. Bring the image nearer and nearer, so that it becomes bigger still. When this image is as big and bold and bright as it can be, mentally say 'yes' very loudly and with great determination.

Clench the fist of your dominant hand as you do so. Repeat this two or three times.

- Now, without allowing the image to shrink or fade, audibly and loudly say 'yes' with as much force and determination as you can clenching the fist of your dominant hand as you do so. Repeat twice more, each time saying 'yes' more loudly than before.

- Now, unclench your fist and allow yourself to relax. As you do so, allow the image to fade. Repeat this exercise at least once a day.

Exercise 16
Picturing your potential self

- Find somewhere comfortable to sit or lie and close your eyes or focus on a fixed point within your line of vision.

- When you are comfortable, begin to count backwards in your mind from 300. If you lose count or if your mind wanders, return to the last number you remember and continue counting downwards.

- Allow yourself to release a little more tension from your body with each number so that as you count downwards you are becoming more and more relaxed.

- When you feel relaxed allow the numbers to fade away.

- Imagine it's a warm sunny day and that you are standing on a sea wall looking out to sea across an empty expanse of sand.

- As you stand there you can feel the sun's rays warming your body and you begin to feel as though you want to lie down.

- Looking to one side you see some steps set in the sea wall. There are 10 in all and they are very steep.

- You move towards the steps and begin to descend them, mentally counting each step, 10, 9, 8 ...

- On step 8 you realise the steps really are very steep and that you are tiring.

- You pause and take a deep breath before descending to step 7, and then the same for step 6, and step 5.

- On reaching the fifth step you realise that the sun's rays are being reflected off the sea wall and you are beginning to feel very warm. Your legs are also beginning to feel heavy with the effort of descending the steps.

- You take a deep breath and, counting as you go, move on to steps 4 and 3.

- On the third step from the bottom you pause again. You are feeling warm and heavy and tired. All you want to do is reach the sand and lie down.

- Breathing in deeply and counting, you step onto step 2, then step 1 and from there you step onto the sand.

- The sand beneath your feet is very fine and soft and it takes a lot of effort to walk through it toward the sea. As you do so your body feels more and more heavy and you feel very tired. All you want to do is lie down.

- After several more strides through the sand you lie down on the sand facing the sea with your arms and legs outstretched.

You can feel the warmth of the sand beneath you and the warmth of the sun from above.

■ As your body is enveloped in this warmth the tension throughout your body eases away, and you begin to relax.

■ As your body relaxes your mind also begins to let go of all tensions, anxieties, preoccupations and concerns.

■ You close your eyes and find that you are looking at a vast empty space. In it appears an image of yourself – the *lazy* you. Notice the appearance of your body, its shape and size and distinguishing features. Notice the way you use your body, and how energetically. Notice the postures you adopt, the movements you make and the speed and fluency of these movements. Be aware of, and accept the features you have been born with and cannot change. Be aware of the features you could change if you chose to.

■ Now, imagine that this image is moving away from you. Allow it to fade into empty space, and spend a few moments contemplating what you have seen and your thoughts and feelings about it.

■ Imagine that another figure appears in your visual space. As it does so you realise that it is an image of your potential self, the very best you can achieve with the body you were born with.

■ Bring it closer so that you can clearly see it and compare it with the image of yourself as you are now.

■ Imagine that the tools you need in order to actualise your potential self are laid out in front of you. They lie between you and it. Be aware of those tools and what they represent. You may see yourself engaging in various activities such as walking, swimming, cycling, housework or dancing, or you may see objects or symbols representing the means by which you can achieve your full potential. Spend some time examining and pondering these images so that you understand them.

■ Then imagine using these tools. Focus attention on the muscles of your body as you do so. Imagine them working more efficiently and effectively. Imagine enjoying working with these tools and working more easily. Then imagine challenging your muscles to work harder, either by using different tools or using the same tools more frequently or for longer. Imagine the effects of doing so on the appearance of your body and your thoughts and feelings about it.

■ See yourself leaner, lighter, stronger, fitter, more supple and toned. Imagine how it feels to actualise your potential. Imagine yourself feeling energetic, active, fully alive, confident and happy. Imagine the lifestyle you can now enjoy. Imagine running forward, arms outstretched, to embrace the new you. See it coming closer and closer, getting bigger and bigger, brighter and bolder. Embrace your full potential. Feel it. Delight in it. Merge with it.

■ As the lazy you is engulfed by the enormity of your full potential look forward to a new future.

■ Feeling energised and excited, you open your eyes and leap to your feet. You turn and look back towards the sea wall, and move swiftly and effortlessly across the sand towards it. Your feet appear hardly to touch the sand.

■ Reaching the steps in the sea wall you begin to climb them easily and quickly, counting as you go, 1, 2, 3, 4, 5, 6, 7, 8, 9, 10.

■ At the top of the sea wall you pause briefly to fix firmly in your mind the image of the new you before walking briskly back to the room you are in, and returning to ordinary awareness.

This exercise uses visualisation to create a positive image to replace a negative one, in this instance, that of being lazy. It is the same technique used in self-hypnosis and can be very powerful in bringing about change. Once created in the mind, this positive image can be summoned at will and used to motivate you to exercise. Practising this simple mind and muscle relaxation technique before exercise will not only inspire you to exercise but will enhance the experience.

Pre-exercise routines of this kind can help anyone reach their personal peak performance – even top athletes commonly prime themselves for action using the same approach. You will find that they help you achieve your own personal exercise goals more easily and enhance your enjoyment of exercise considerably. Imagining that you can now stretch yourself physically is an excellent preparation for the exercises in Chapter 6.

CHAPTER 6

STRETCH YOURSELF

Watch any cat or dog and you'll see that it stretches instinctively and naturally before lying down to sleep. After a period of inactivity it will stretch in order to prepare itself for movement. Doing so relaxes the muscles and helps to prevent undue strain in the transition from activity to inactivity and vice versa. It also promotes flexibility and suppleness. Stretching serves the same functions in humans but when humans become sedentary they are less inclined to stretch spontaneously.

Muscles tighten because of nervous tension. This wastes energy and creates muscle fatigue that is felt as aches and pains and tiredness. Muscle-stretching exercises promote both mental and physical fitness, achieve a better balance of body and mind, and help people feel good about themselves.

Stretch-based relaxation training uses stretching exercises as an alternative to the tension-release methods of progressive relaxation. It avoids the interruption of the relaxation process by muscle tensing and has been found to be effective in decreasing muscle tension and activation, and also has potential for stress management. Sports scientists now recognise that fitness can be improved with certain kinds of stretching: ballistic or movement stretches, static stretches such as those used in yoga, isometric or flex and relax stretches, and passive stretches where a joint is held in a certain position and pressure applied to it. These kinds of stretching promote flexibility and are used in fitness training.

Stretching has many benefits, both physical and psychological. By stretching muscles we allow them to relax to their full length so that the full range of the muscle is used instead of remaining in a semi-contracted, tight, mid-range state. This enables freer and easier movement and increases the range of motion. Stretching also improves circulation and warms the muscles. Many injuries occur because tense, cold muscles are made to work. Stretching beforehand signals to muscles that they are about to be used and helps to prevent strain and injury resulting from sudden movement. Stretching therefore relaxes the body, helps it move better and improves its ability to cope with physical tasks. If repeated regularly and frequently, it builds the foundation for fitness and gets the body in shape.

Psychologically, stretching muscles calms the mind, increases confidence and the ability to cope with tasks. By focusing attention on the muscles it develops muscle sense and puts you more in touch with your body. Perhaps most importantly stretching feels good and promotes feelings of enhanced pleasure and well-being. It helps you enjoy movement.

Even if you hate exercise and would never dream of setting foot in a gym, you can make stretching part of your daily routine and gain all the benefits. If you don't, you are likely to be unbalanced, quite literally. Most of us, whether we are aware of it or not, are lopsided. We favour one side of our body over the other for carrying bags, lifting heavy items, and holding the telephone. Over time this causes our bodies to become asymmetrical and results in muscular imbalances that have potentially serious consequences for the spine, contributing to pain in the neck, back and limbs.

Sitting at a computer for more than an hour each day can have dramatic effects on your body and your life. Pressure on the nerves of the neck can result in migraine, blurred vision, and numbness, pain or tingling in the fingers. Nerve compression in the neck and upper back can also be a contributory factor in asthma and bronchial conditions, while pressure on the nerves of the middle and lower back can contribute significantly to stomach and bowel problems respectively. Holding a telephone to the ear causes the neck muscles to stiffen and cupping the phone between the ear and shoulder shortens the muscles on one side of the neck and compresses the nerves. These problems can be prevented by changing habitual patterns, for instance, avoiding cupping the phone to the ear and alternating the ear used, and not remaining seated for long periods without movement.

The growing concern about deep vein thrombosis resulting from long haul air flights has highlighted the potentially damaging and even deadly consequences of sitting in one position for considerable lengths of time without moving. The recommended guidelines for reducing the risk of this condition include moving the body and limbs frequently, and stretching the body and limbs regularly if this is not possible. So, developing the habit of stretching regularly doesn't simply enhance fitness and well-being. It can save your life.

HOW TO STRETCH

Stretching is easy to do but it is important to do it correctly. The correct way is a relaxed, sustained stretch with your attention focused on the muscles that you are working. Performing short, jerky or bouncing movements or stretching to the point of pain is incorrect because it triggers the stretch reflex that protects muscles by contracting them. Stretching expert Bob Anderson recommends a three-stage process when you stretch. This begins with the *easy* stretch, which reduces muscular tightness and readies the muscles for the second stage, *developmental* stretch, which fine-tunes muscles and increases flexibility. If repeated regularly over time this enables you to go beyond your present limits and achieve naturally, without trying, the *drastic* stretch, or the elongation potential of your muscles.

The easy stretch is achieved by stretching to the point where you can feel a mild tension. When you achieve this, relax and hold the stretch for 10–30 seconds (a slow count to 20). The feeling of tension should subside as you hold the position. If it doesn't, ease the stretch slightly and find a degree of tension that is comfortable. After the easy stretch, move slowly, without jerking or bouncing, into the developmental stretch by moving just a fraction further until you again feel a mild tension. Hold this position for 10–30 seconds. The tension should diminish. If it doesn't, ease off slightly until you find a position that is comfortable. In both stages, silently count the seconds for each stretch to ensure you hold the tension long enough. Over time you will be able to stretch by the way it feels not by counting. Throughout the stretch your breathing should be slow, rhythmical and controlled.

Remember:

- Stretch only within your limitations. Do not overstretch and do not compete if exercising with others. You risk injury if you do so. Everyone differs in the degree of flexibility they possess. Increased flexibility comes with practice. The more familiar you become with the exercises the longer you will be able to hold each stretch and the more flexible you will become.

- Always work within your comfort zone. Only apply gentle pressure when stretching and never force any movement.

- Breathe out as you stretch, then maintain slow and relaxed breathing while you stay in the stretched position.

- Never hold your breath.

- Stop if you experience pain.

STRETCHING EXERCISES

The following exercises include stretches for each part of the body. They can be used to warm up before more strenuous exercise and to cool down afterwards. However, stretching can be done any time you feel like it. Stretching soon after you rise in the morning will help you prepare for the day's activity. Stretching during the day will help you to release muscular tension, particularly if you have been sitting or standing for a long time, or feel stiff. You can stretch when standing in queues or sitting in your car during traffic jams, when watching television, listening to music or the radio, lying on a sofa, a beach, or in bed. Stretching before you retire at night or when in bed can help you relax and sleep well.

Because you can stretch when standing, sitting or lying down, the exercises that follow are grouped in those categories. Each group of stretches constitutes a complete body workout (standing, pages 72–84; sitting, pages 84–97; lying down, 97–110). These are followed by three speedy stretches (pages 110–112) – one standing, one sitting and one lying down – which provide a full body stretch for those occasions when you don't have time to do the full set of stretches for every part of the body. On pages 112–120 are specific exercises that can be performed when you are sitting at a desk or computer, in a car or aeroplane, or after a long telephone call.

STANDING STRETCHES

Exercise 17
Supported calf stretch

Stretches the lower leg, heel, and ankle joint.

- Face something you can lean against for support such as a wall or a secure post.

- Stand a little distance from it with both feet pointing directly forward, not outward.

- Rest your forearms against the support.

- Rest your forehead on the back of your hands.

- Bend one of your knees and move your foot slightly nearer the support.

- Keep the back leg straight and the foot flat to the floor.

- Without changing the position of your feet, slowly move your hips forward.

■ When you feel the stretch in the calf muscles of your lower leg, hold for 20 seconds.

■ Then increase the stretch slightly into a developmental stretch and hold for 20 seconds.

■ Stretch the other leg in the same way.

A variation of this exercise is to face a wall, standing a metre from it. Lean towards it supporting the weight of your body with outstretched arms. While keeping the feet pointed directly forward, lower both heels to the floor. Move one foot closer to the wall, bending it as you do so. When you feel the stretch in the calf of the rear leg, hold it for 20 seconds. Release and change legs. The stretch can be developed by moving slightly further backwards.

Exercise 18
Free-standing calf stretch

Stretches the lower leg muscles, heel and ankle joint.

■ Stand with one foot forward and one foot back, with both feet pointing directly forward and not turned outward.

■ Bend the knee of the leading leg and allow your weight to come forward over that leg.

■ Keep your back leg straight and the heel to the ground.

■ When you feel the stretch in the calf region of the back leg, hold for 20 seconds.

■ Increase the stretch slightly and hold it for 20 seconds.

■ Change the leading leg and repeat.

Exercise 19
Standing thigh stretch

This stretches the thighs and the hip flexor muscles.

- Either hold on to a wall or other support, or stand free and in balance.

- Flex one knee and lift the foot of that leg towards the buttock.

- Grasp that foot with one or both hands.

- Gently pull the heel of the foot in towards the buttock, at the same time pushing the hips forward.

- Keep the thigh pointing down and your knees together.

- Keep the knee of the supporting leg slightly bent.

- Don't allow the back to curve excessively.

- When you feel the stretch in your thigh, hold for 20 seconds.

- Develop the stretch by gently moving the hip further forward and holding the position for 20 seconds.

Exercise 20
Hamstring stretch

Stretches the muscles at the backs of the thighs.

- Stand with one foot in front of the other with the leading leg straight, the back leg bent at the knee and both feet facing forward. Do not turn the feet out.

- Bend forward from your hips, supporting the weight of your body on the arms by resting your hands on the thigh of the bent leg.

- When you feel a gentle stretch on the back of the thigh of the front straight leg hold it for 20 seconds.

- Develop the stretch by slowly flexing the foot of the leading leg. Keep the heel to the floor. Hold for 20 seconds.

- To develop the stretch further, move your arms from the thigh and hold the flexed foot. Hold for 20 seconds.

- The stretch can be developed even further by letting go of the flexed foot and touching the floor to either side of the foot with your hands.

Exercise 21
Adductor stretch

Stretches the inner thigh muscles.

- Stand with legs fairly wide apart.

- Turn one foot slightly to one side, bend the knee of that leg and slowly lean toward it. Do not lean too far as this will place excessive strain on the knee joint.

- Keep your body facing forward. Do not turn to the side.

- Keep the other leg straight and the foot of that leg pointing forward and flat to the floor.

- When you feel a gentle stretch on the inner thigh of the straight leg, hold it for 20 seconds.

- Develop the stretch by leaning slightly further toward the bent knee and hold for 20 seconds.

- Repeat with the other leg.

Exercise 22
Hip rotation

Releases tension in the hip joints.

- Stand upright, your feet hip-width apart.
- Place your arms on your hips and very slowly rotate your hips to one side five times.
- Repeat, moving your hips in the opposite direction.

Exercise 23
Lower back stretch

Stretches the buttocks and lower back muscles.

- Stand with feet together.
- Tighten the muscles of your buttocks.
- Breathe in.
- Place your hands on your buttocks and push forward, arching your back and looking directly upwards as you do.
- Do not bend your knees.
- Hold the position for 20 seconds.
- Breathe out as you return to the upright position.

Exercise 24
Standing side reaches

Stretches the waist and side muscles.

- Stand with your feet wider apart than your hips, your knees slightly bent and your arms down by your sides, hands resting on your thighs.

- Breathe in and raise one arm, keeping your shoulder blades down in your back for as long as possible.

- Keep your neck and upper shoulder relaxed.

- Don't move your arm forward or back.

- Don't look up or down.

- Finish the movement with the palm of your hand facing inwards.

- Breathe out and as you do so slide your other arm down the outside of your thigh.

- When you feel the stretch in your side, breathe in as you return to an upright position.

- Repeat five times on each side.

Exercise 25
Waist twists

This stretches the rear abdominal muscles.

- Stand upright with your feet hip-width apart.

- Raise both arms, with elbows loosely bent and hands relaxed.

- Keeping your lower body still and your hip bones and head facing forward, gently twist to one side.

- Hold the position for 20 seconds. Repeat five times.

- Repeat on the other side.

- Do not twist your hips.

Exercise 26
Side bends

Stretches the oblique muscles.

- Stand upright with your feet hip-width apart and arms hanging loosely at your sides.

- Without bending the knees or turning the head, gently bend to one side so that your arm slides down towards the knee.

- When you feel a stretch in your sides, hold the position for 20 seconds.

- To develop the stretch, allow your hand to slide further down your leg and hold for 20 seconds.

- Repeat five times.

- Change side and repeat five times.

Exercise 27
Overhead side bends

Stretches the muscles of the outer arms, shoulders and ribs.

- Stand upright, your feet hip-width apart and facing forward.

- Extend your arms above your head and clasp your hands together.

- Stretch the arms upward and slightly backwards, breathing in as you do.

- Hold the stretch for 20 seconds.

- Ease the stretch slightly, breathing out as you do.

- Stretch upward again, and lean to one side, breathing in as you do.

- Feel an easy stretch in your side and chest, and hold for 20 seconds.

- Develop the stretch by leaning slightly further to that side, and hold for 20 seconds.

- Breathe out and change sides.

Exercise 28
Scapular squeeze

Stretches the shoulder blades.

- Stand with feet parallel, hip-width apart.

- Bend your knees so that they are directly over your feet.

- Lean forward from your hips as though you are skiing downhill.

- Keep your head, neck and back in a straight line.

- Keep your neck and back free of tension.

- Take your arms behind you at the sides with the palms of your hands facing down as though you are making a downhill ski jump.

- Breathe out and slide your shoulder blades down your back.

- Squeeze your shoulder blades together.

- Squeeze your arms together so that the thumbs of your hands meet.

- Breathe in and hold this stretch for 20 seconds.

- Breathe out as you release the stretch.

- Repeat five times before returning to an upright position.

Exercise 29
Shoulder stretch

This stretches the muscles of the upper arms and the top of the shoulders.

- Stand facing forward, feet hip-width apart and knees slightly bent.

- Extend one arm above the head and bend the elbow, placing the hand down behind the neck and between the shoulder blades.

- With the hand of the other arm hold the elbow.

- Slowly and gently stretch the elbow by pushing it downwards behind your head.

- Hold the position for 20 seconds.

- Stretch the elbow of the other arm in the same way.

You can vary this exercise by standing with knees slightly bent; as you gently pull your elbow behind your head, bend your hips to the side. When you feel the stretch, hold it for 20 seconds and repeat on the other side.

Exercise 30
Upper back stretch

Stretches the muscles of the upper arms and shoulders.

■ Stand with legs hip-width apart and knees slightly bent.

■ Stretch both of your arms forward and link the fingers of your hands.

■ Turn your palms outward.

■ Push forward with your arms and allow the back to curl forward.

■ When you feel the stretch across your upper back and shoulders hold for 20 seconds.

■ Develop the stretch by pushing your arms slightly further forward and hold for 20 seconds.

Exercise 31
Chest stretch

Stretches the chest and front of the shoulders.

■ Stand with legs hip-width apart and knees slightly bent. Look straight ahead, not down.

■ Stretch both arms out behind your back and link the fingers of your hands.

■ Pull your arms back until you feel the stretch across your chest and the front of your shoulders.

■ Hold for 20 seconds.

■   Develop the stretch by raising your arms towards the shoulders slightly, and hold for 20 seconds.

Exercise 32
Arms stretch

Stretches the muscles of the back and arms.

■   Stand with your feet together.

■   Take a deep in-breath and hold it.

■   Entwine your fingers behind your back.

■   Tighten the muscles of your buttocks.

■   Pull both arms downward towards your heels, arching your back as you do so and looking up.

■   Hold for 20 seconds.

■   Breathe out and return to normal position.

Exercise 33
Standing shoulder circles

Releases tension in the shoulders.

■   Stand upright breathing normally.

■   Starting the movement from your chest, rotate your shoulders in backward circles.

■   Keep your head and neck relaxed, lengthening your neck as though your head is being gently pulled upwards.

■   Repeat five times.

■ Repeat five times rotating your shoulders in forward circles.

■ When you have done this, bend your elbows and, breathing normally, circle your arms forward and backward. Do this five times in each direction.

■ Then hold your arms forward in a natural curve with the elbows only slightly crooked.

■ Circle backward moving the entire arm.

■ Repeat five times before circling the arms forward five times.

Exercise 34
Sideways head roll

Stretches the muscles of the neck and will help to release joint stiffness by dispersing calcium deposits that often settle on joint surfaces.

■ Stand comfortably, head upright and looking straight ahead.

■ Bend your head forward so that your chin touches your chest.

■ Very slowly roll your head in the direction of your right shoulder, ensuring that your chin and lower jaw maintain contact with your chest and shoulders throughout the rotation.

■ Repeat five times and then change direction.

Exercise 35
Full head roll

Stretches the muscles of the neck and face.

■ Stand comfortably, head upright and looking straight ahead.

- Very slowly roll your head in a full circle, keeping your back straight.

- If at any point your neck feels stiff, pause and stretch the area that feels tight.

- Roll your head slowly in one direction and then the other.

- When you have done this, slowly move your head forward stretching your chin toward your neck. Hold this position for 20 seconds.

- Slowly move your head upwards and back, stretching your neck.

- Hold for 20 seconds.

- Do not strain.

- Repeat three times.

SEATED STRETCHES

To be performed when sitting on the floor.

Exercise 36
Seated lower leg stretch

Stretches the muscles of the lower legs and backs of the knees.

- Sit with legs straight in front of you.

- Keep your head up, looking forward, and your back straight.

- Slowly bring both feet into an upright position.

- Hold them in this position for 20 seconds before gently stretching the feet forward as far as you can, pointing the toes as you do so.

- Hold this position for 20 seconds.

- Repeat five times.

Exercise 37
Seated hamstring stretch

Stretches the entire spine and the muscles along the back of the thighs and behind the knees.

- Sit comfortably on the floor with legs straight, feet upright and heels about 15cm apart.

- Slowly bend forward from the hips, lengthening your neck.

- Don't allow your head to dip or your hips to roll back.

- Hold this easy stretch for 20 seconds.

Exercise 38
Alternate hamstring stretch

Stretches the muscles of the lower back and the inner thighs.

- Sit comfortably on the floor with one leg forward in a straight line from your hip and the foot relaxed, and the other leg bent so that the sole of its foot rests against the inside of your knee.

- Breathe out and gently lean forward, resting your arms in front of you.

- Keep your neck long and your shoulder blades down into your back.

- Take 10 breaths in this position.

- Breathe out and slowly return to an upright position.

- Repeat with the other leg.

Exercise 39
Groin stretch

Stretches the inside of the upper thighs.

- Sit comfortably on the floor.

- Place the soles of your feet together and your hands around your feet and toes.

- Keep the heels a comfortable distance from your body.

- Gently pull the upper body forward until you feel an easy stretch in your groin area.

- Hold for 20 seconds.

- To develop the stretch lean slightly further forward and hold for 20 seconds.

Exercise 40
Adductor stretch

Stretches the inner thighs and spine.

- Sit comfortably on the floor with your legs in front of you a comfortable distance apart and your toes pointed forward.

- Do not force your knees down to the floor.

- Rest your hands on your knees.

- Breathe in and lift the spine out of the hips, lengthening upwards through your backbone as you do so.

- Breathe out, tighten the muscles of your abdomen, and with your chin tucked in, slowly curl downward aiming the top of your head towards the centre of your stomach, allowing your arms to reach forward as you do so.

■ Breathing normally, inch your hands forward as far as you can.

■ If you can, press your knees to the floor.

■ Hold this position for 10 breaths.

■ After 10 breaths slowly return to an upright position, bringing your head up last.

■ Repeat three times.

Exercise 41
Spinal stretch

Lengthens the spine along its length and the inner thigh muscles and releases tension from the shoulders.

■ Sit comfortably on the floor with your knees bent, the soles of your feet together and your head up looking forward. (Sit with your buttocks and back aligned against a wall if you wish).

■ Do not bring the feet too close to your body.

■ Breathe out and as you do so gently tighten the muscles of your abdomen.

■ Lift your body upwards from your hips and slowly lean forward placing your hands around your ankles, allowing your arms to rest across your upper thighs.

■ Allow your neck to lengthen and your shoulder blades to relax down into your back.

- Remain in this position and take 10 breaths.

- After 10 breaths, breathe out and slowly bring your head upward and return to normal.

Exercise 42
Spinal twist

Flexes the spine and relieves tension in the lower back.

- Sit on the floor with your legs in front of you and the backs of your heels on the floor and the feet upright.

- Keep your back straight but not too stiff, as if your head is being pulled slightly in an upward direction.

- Bend your right leg and lift it over the left leg at the knee.

- Support your upper body by placing it behind you, palm down, in alignment with your spine.

- Avoid putting your weight on this hand.

- Place your right hand on the floor beside your left thigh.

- Take a deep breath, and as you breathe out, twist your upper body to the left, leading with your head but allowing your shoulders to make the rotation.

- Keep your buttocks and legs firmly on the ground.

- Hold for 20 seconds.

- Breathe in and return to the starting position.

- Breathe out and repeat the movement, trying to twist a little further than before.

- Hold for 20 seconds.

- Breathe in and return to the starting position.

- Repeat this movement with the other leg.

- Ensure that throughout the exercise your movements are slow and smooth. Do not jerk.

Exercise 43
Seated waist twist

Stretches the muscles of the lower abdomen.

- Sit on the floor with legs outstretched in front of you or crossed, whichever is more comfortable.

- Keep your back straight and your head upright looking straight ahead.

- Raise both arms, with elbows loosely bent and hands relaxed.

- With your hip bones and head facing forward, gently twist to one side.

- Hold the position for 20 seconds. Repeat five times.

- Repeat on the other side.

Exercise 44
Upper body stretch

Stretches the area between the shoulders and around the arms.

- Sit on the floor facing a wall.

- Cross your legs.

- Place the palms of your hands flat against the wall above you and wider than your shoulders.

- Keep the angle to your elbows open and your shoulder blades down into your back.

- Breathe out, tightening the muscles of your abdomen as you do so.

- Keeping the abdominal muscles tight but breathing normally, lean towards the wall.

- Hold the stretch for 20 seconds.

- Return to an upright position.

- Repeat five times.

- To develop the stretch, sit further away from the wall.

Exercise 45
Shoulder twist

Stretches the muscles of the shoulder and upper body.

- Sit comfortably cross-legged with your right side against a wall.

- Place your hands on the wall, out to the sides and at shoulder height.

- Breathe out, tightening the muscles of your abdomen as you do so and slowly turn your upper body towards the wall, pushing a little against your right hand.

- Hold the stretch for 20 seconds.

- Repeat three times.

■ Turn around so that your left side is against the wall and repeat the stretch three times, pushing your left hand against the wall as you do so.

Exercise 46
Seated overhead side bends

Stretches the muscles of the outer arms, shoulders and ribs.

■ Sit on the floor with legs outstretched in front of you or crossed, whichever is more comfortable.

■ Keep your back straight and your head upright looking straight ahead.

■ Extend your arms above your head and clasp your hands together.

■ Hold the stretch for 20 seconds.

■ Ease the stretch slightly, breathing out as you do so.

■ Stretch upwards again, and lean to one side, breathing in as you do so.

■ Feel an easy stretch in your side and chest and hold for the count of 10.

■ Develop the stretch by leaning slightly further to that side and hold for 20 seconds.

■ Breathe out and repeat the exercise on the other side.

Exercise 47
Seated shoulder stretch

Stretches the triceps muscle and the top of the shoulders.

- Sit with your legs outstretched in front of you or crossed, whichever is more comfortable.

- Keep your back straight, your head upright, looking forward.

- Extend one arm above the head and bend the elbow, placing the hand down behind the neck and between the shoulder blades.

- With the hand of the other arm hold the elbow.

- Slowly and gently stretch the elbow by pulling it downwards behind your head.

- Hold the position for 20 seconds.

- Stretch the elbow of the other arm in the same way.

Exercise 48
Seated upper back stretch

Stretches upper back and shoulders.

- Sit with your legs outstretched in front of you or crossed, whichever is more comfortable.

- Stretch both of your arms forward and link the fingers of your hands.

- Turn your hands palm outward.

- Push forward with your arms and allow your back to curl forward.

- When you feel an easy stretch across your upper back and shoulders hold for 20 seconds.

■   Develop the stretch by pushing your arms slightly further forward and hold for 20 seconds.

Exercise 49
Seated chest stretch

Stretches the chest and the front of the shoulders.

■   Sit on the floor with your legs outstretched in front of you or crossed, whichever is more comfortable.

■   Keep your back straight and head upright, looking forward. Don't look down.

■   Stretch both arms out behind your back and link the fingers of your hands.

■   Pull your arm back until you feel an easy stretch across your chest and the front of your shoulders.

■   Hold for 20 seconds.

■   Develop the stretch by raising the arms towards the shoulders slightly and hold for 20 seconds.

Exercise 50
Seated arm stretch

Stretches the muscles of the outer and inner arms.

■   Sit on the floor with legs outstretched in front of you, or crossed, whichever is more comfortable.

■   Keep your back straight, head up and look straight ahead.

■   Extend both arms out to the sides at shoulder height.

- Turn your hands upward so that your palms are facing away from you.

- Gently stretch the arms to the side as if pushing your palms as far away from your body as you can.

- When you feel the stretch along both arms hold for 20 seconds.

- When you have done this, slowly rotate the arms 20 times in each direction.

Exercise 51
Seated scapular squeeze

Releases tension between the shoulder blades.

- Sit with feet outstretched in front of you or crossed, whichever is more comfortable.

- Keep your back straight and your head up, looking straight ahead.

- Lean forward from the hips, keeping your head neck and back in a straight line.

- Look at a spot on the floor in front of you.

- Keeping your neck and back free of tension, take your arms behind you to the sides with the palms of your hands facing up.

- Breathe out and slide your shoulder blades down your back.

- Squeeze your shoulder blades together and also your arms so that your thumbs meet.

- Breathe in and hold for 20 seconds.

- Breathe out as you release the stretch.

- Repeat five times before returning to an upright position.

Exercise 52
Seated shoulder circles

Releases tension in the shoulder joints.

- Sit upright, with your neck and back straight, lengthening your neck as if your head is being pulled gently upwards.

- Breathing normally and keeping your neck relaxed, rotate your shoulders backward in circles, starting the movement from your chest.

- Repeat five times.

- Now rotate your shoulders forward and repeat five times.

- Having done so, bend both elbows and, breathing normally, circle your arms backwards five times, then forwards five times.

- Hold your arms forward in a natural curve with your elbows only slightly crooked and circle backwards, moving the whole arm.

- Repeat five times before circling the arm forward five times.

Exercise 53
Seated sideways head roll

Releases tension in the neck.

- Sit on the floor with your legs outstretched in front of you or crossed, whichever is more comfortable.

- Keep your back straight, head upright and look straight ahead.

- Bend your head forward so that your chin touches your chest.

- Very slowly and smoothly roll your head in the direction of one of your shoulders ensuring that your chin and lower jaw maintain contact with your chest and shoulder throughout the rotation.

- Repeat five times and then change direction.

Exercise 54
Seated full head roll

Breaks down calcium deposits in the neck.

- Sit on the floor with your legs straight in front of you or crossed, whichever is more comfortable.

- Keep your back straight and your head up and look straight ahead.

- Very slowly roll your head in a full circle.

- If at any point your neck feels stiff, pause and stretch the area that feels tight.

- Roll your head slowly and smoothly in one direction and then the other.

- When you have done this, slowly move your head forward stretching your chin in towards your neck.

- Hold for 20 seconds.

- Slowly move your head upwards and back, stretching your neck.

- Hold for 20 seconds.

- Do not strain.

- Repeat three times.

LYING STRETCHES

To be performed lying down, preferably on a firm surface. You may want to support your head with a folded towel or thin cushion.

Exercise 55
Foot rotation

Loosens the ankle joints.

- Lie on your back with your knees bent, your feet hip-width apart and parallel.

- Bring one knee up towards your chest so that it is directly above your hip.

- Circle the foot of the raised leg slowly in a complete circle five times.

- Change the direction of the movement and repeat five times.

- Move only the foot. Do not allow the leg or pelvis to move.

- Change leg and repeat the movement five times in each direction before returning to the starting position.

Exercise 56
Knee circles

Maintains hip mobility.

- Lie on your back with your knees bent, your feet hip-width apart and parallel.

- Bring one knee up towards your chest so that it is directly above your hip.

- Breathing normally, gently rotate the bent leg.

- Do not move the torso or allow it to rock from side to side

- Repeat the movement five times, first in one direction, then the other.

- Change leg and rotate it five times in each direction before returning to the starting position.

Exercise 57
Leg circles

Maintains hip mobility and stretches and tones the thigh muscles.

- Lie on your back with knees bent, hip-width apart and parallel.

- Straighten one leg and raise it in the air as near to vertical as you can without strain or pain.

- Straighten the leg as fully as you can and when you can easily straighten the leg, flex the foot.

- Keep your other foot on the floor, with the knee bent.

■ Without moving your hips or lifting your lower back from the ground, rotate the leg slowly in a circle, five times in one direction, then five times in the opposite direction, before returning to the starting position.

Exercise 58
Hamstring stretch

Stretches the muscles at the back of the legs that flex and bend the knee.

■ Lie on your back with your knees bent, feet flat on the floor and hip-width apart.

■ Bend one knee towards your chest

■ Hold the lower leg gently and straighten the leg into the air.

■ Flex the foot downward towards your face.

■ If you can, fully straighten the leg.

■ When you feel a stretch along the length of your leg hold the stretch for 20 seconds, breathing normally.

■ Relax the leg by gently bending it.

■ Repeat five times with each leg.

Exercise 59
Hip flexor stretch

Stretches the *psoas* or hip flexor muscles.

■ Lie on your back with your knees bent and feet flat on the floor.

- Breathe out and as you do so draw one of your knees to your chest.

- Breathe in and clasp the leg below the knee (or behind the lower part of the thigh).

- Holding on to the leg, breathe out as you extend your other leg along the floor.

- Do not arch your back. Keep it on the floor.

- Breathe in as you return the leg to the starting position.

- Repeat with the other leg.

- To develop the stretch as you bring your knee to your chest, bring your head forward to touch your knee, breathing out slowly as you do so.

- Lower your head to the floor slowly, keeping your chin in towards your neck and breathing in.

- Breathe out and straighten the leg.

- Repeat five times with each leg.

Exercise 60
Back twist

Flexes the spine along its length.

- Lie on your back, with legs outstretched and parallel.

- Extend both arms out to the sides at shoulder level.

- Keeping your feet on the floor, slowly bend both of your knees.

- Take a deep breath and turn your head to one side so that you are looking at the back of your hand, and as you do so, slowly lower your knees to the floor on the opposite side.

- Keep your knees together and your shoulders to the floor.

- Do not rush the movement and do not allow the knees to drop to the floor. Lower them gently.

- Hold for 20 seconds.

- Repeat the exercise turning your head to the other side and lowering your knees in the opposite direction.

- Repeat two or three times on each side.

Exercise 61
Pelvic lift

Maintains the flexibility of the spine.

- Lie on your back with your feet flat on the floor about 30cm from your buttocks, parallel and hip-width apart.

- Keep your arms at your sides, slightly away from your body.

- Breathe out and raise your spine off the floor, raising your pelvis as high as you can.

- Do not arch your back.

- Keep your neck straight and relaxed.

- Breathe in and hold the position for 20 seconds.

- Breathe out and slowly lower your back to the floor, feeling each vertebra touch the floor as you do so.

- Repeat five times.

Exercise 62
Shoulder blade pull

Releases tension in the shoulders.

- Lie flat with knees bent and feet flat on the floor.
- Place your hands behind your head and interlace your fingers.
- Breathe out as you pull your shoulder blades together towards the centre of your spine.
- Hold for 20 seconds.
- Relax.
- Repeat five times.

Exercise 63
Shoulder hug

Stretches shoulders and upper arms.

- Lie flat on your back with knees bent and feet flat on the floor.
- Cross your arms over your chest with the right arm over the left so that your hands are touching the opposite shoulder.
- Breathe out and hug yourself.
- Hold for 20 seconds.
- Unfold your arms and return to the starting position.
- Repeat five times.

■ Don't shorten your neck as you hug yourself.

Exercise 64
Chest press

Releases tension in the chest.

■ Lie flat with your knees bent and feet flat on the floor.

■ Interlace your fingers and place them palms upward on your chest.

■ Breathe out and press your hands upward, straightening your elbows and releasing your shoulder blades.

■ Hold for 20 seconds.

■ Breathe in and lower your arms toward the floor behind your head.

■ Breathe out, release your hands and circle your arms down towards your outer thighs.

■ Repeat five times.

Exercise 65
Shoulder drops

Releases tension in the upper body.

■ Lie on your back with knees bent and your feet hip-width apart and flat on the floor.

■ Straighten both arms and raise them directly upwards in a vertical line with your shoulders.

- Breathe in as you reach one arm further upwards, allowing the shoulder blade to lift from the floor.

- Stretch the arm right through to the fingertips.

- Breathe out as you allow the entire shoulder to lower to the floor.

- Repeat with the other arm and then 10 times with each arm alternately.

- Return to the starting position with arms raised above the head.

- Breathe in and reach one arm across in the direction of the opposite knee, allowing the shoulder to lift from the ground.

- Breathe out as you allow the entire shoulder to return to the floor.

- Repeat with the other arm and then 10 times with each arm alternately.

Exercise 66
Chin press

Stretches and releases tension in the neck.

- Lie flat on your back with your arms relaxed by your sides.

- Breathe out as you gently press your chin downward into your neck so that the back of your neck is lengthening and pressing into the floor.

- Hold the position for 20 seconds

- Breathe in and relax.

■   Repeat five times.

Exercise 67
Neck twist

Loosens the neck muscles.

■   Lie flat on your back, arms relaxed by your sides.

■   Keeping your spine straight along its length from neck to lower back, breathe in and rotate your head directly to one side and place your ear on/towards the floor.

■   Hold for 20 seconds.

■   Return to centre.

■   Breathe out and rotate your head to the other side so as to place your ear on/towards the floor.

■   Hold for 20 seconds.

■   Repeat three times on each side.

Exercise 68
Head roll

Promotes flexibility in the neck and releases tension from it.

■   Lie on your back with knees bent and feet flat on the ground.

■   Slowly drop your chin onto your chest.

■   Keep your shoulder blades flat to the floor.

■   Gently roll your chin in a quarter circle to one side, eventually bringing it to look directly over the shoulder.

- Slowly reverse the movement until you are looking directly over the opposite shoulder.

- Repeat five times.

For the following exercises you need to roll over on to your stomach.

Exercise 69
Buttock squeeze

Releases tension in the seat muscles.

- Lie face down with your feet hip-width apart and parallel.

- Create a diamond shape with your arms by opening your elbows and relaxing your shoulder blades.

- Place one hand over the other.

- Rest your forehead on the back of the uppermost hand.

- Breathe out and as you do so tighten your buttocks, allowing the legs to draw together and the heels of the feet to touch.

- Hold the position for 20 seconds.

- Relax and repeat five times.

Exercise 70
Upper back stretch

Stretches shoulder blades and muscles of the chest.

- Lie face down with your legs together and parallel and your toes pointed.

- Place your arms down by your sides with the palms of your hands facing your body.

- Allow the neck to lengthen.

- Breathe in and lengthen through the spine and the top of the head.

- Breathe out and pull your shoulder blades down and into your back, lifting your upper body off the floor as you do so and lengthening your fingers away from you and down towards your feet.

- Keep the neck long. Do not allow it to shorten.

- Keep looking down at the floor throughout the movement.

- Squeeze your inner thighs together but keep your feet on the floor.

- Breathe in and hold the position for 20 seconds.

- Breathe out and slowly lower your upper body to the floor.

- Relax and repeat three times.

Exercise 71
Abdominal stretch

Stretches the muscles of the upper abdomen.

- Lie flat on the floor face down, legs slightly apart and parallel, with feet pointed.

- Place the palms of your hands flat on the floor beside your shoulders.

- Breathe in and as you do so lift your chest up and look up.

- Do not overstretch your neck by raising your chin upwards.

- When you feel the stretch below your ribcage hold the position for 20 seconds.

- Breathe out and gently return to the starting position, placing your forehead on the floor.

- Repeat five times.

Exercise 72
Limb stretch

Flexes the spine along its length, the abdominal muscles, and muscles of the arms and legs.

- Lie face downwards with your feet hip-width apart and slightly turned out at the hips.

- Extend your arms in front of your head, placing them slightly wider than your shoulders.

- Keep your shoulder blades down in your back.

- Breathe out and as you do so raise one arm and the opposite leg approximately 5cm from the ground.

- Do not twist your pelvis. Keep both hip joints on the floor.

- Gently stretch the arm and leg away from the centre of your body as far as you can without overreaching.

- Keep the elbows slightly bent.

- When you feel that you are fully stretched from the tip of your fingers to the tip of the toes on the opposite foot hold the position for 20 seconds.

■ Breathe in and slowly lower your limbs to the ground.

■ Breathe out and repeat the action with the opposite arm and leg.

■ Repeat five times.

Exercise 73
Spinal curl

Maintains mobility in the spine.

■ Kneel on all fours with your hands a little wider than shoulder-width apart and underneath your shoulders, fingers forward, and your knees in line with your hips and your toes stretched out.

■ Breathe out and arch the spine up, tightening your lower abdominal muscles as you do so.

■ Keep your chin in towards your chest and your head and neck relaxed.

■ Breathe in as you hold the position for 20 seconds.

■ Breathe out and lower your spine back to the starting position, bringing your neck and head into line with it as you do so.

■ Repeat five times.

Exercise 74
Back stretch

Stretches the muscles of the upper back and shoulders.

- Kneel on all fours, knees hip-width apart and directly under your hips and hands slightly wider apart than your shoulders.

- Bring your feet together so that your toes touch.

- Breathe out and slowly lean back towards your buttocks.

- Do not raise your head or hands.

- Sit on your feet, not between them.

- Relax in this position with the arms extended forward.

- Take 10 breaths.

- Breathe in and gently draw your body backwards so that your hands rest on your thighs.

- From this position slowly stand up bringing your head up last.

SPEEDY STRETCHES

If you haven't time for a fully integrated series of body stretches, you will benefit from the following full body exercises.

Exercise 75
Standing full body stretch

Stand up straight, your feet hip-width apart and flat on the ground, with your arms by your sides.

- Keep your head up and look straight ahead.

- Loosely link the fingers of each hand in front of your body.

- Breathe out and raise your hands above your head, stretching out the fingers as far as they will reach.

- Allow the neck to lengthen as though your head is being gently pulled upwards.

- If you can, slowly rise on tiptoe and when you feel the stretch throughout your entire body, breathe out and slowly lower your feet to the ground and bring your arms to rest by your sides.

- Don't allow your arms to drop. Lower them in a slow, graceful and controlled movement.

- Repeat three times.

Exercise 76
Seated full body stretch (requires a good deal of flexibility)

- Sit on the floor with legs outstretched in front of you, knees very straight and feet together.

- Breathe in and stretch your arms above your head.

- Breathe out very slowly and smoothly bend forwards from your hips, not the waist, to grasp your toes (if this is difficult, hold your ankles, lower legs or knees).

- Keep your legs straight.

- Continue to bend forward and down slowly, aiming to touch your knees with your forehead.

- Hold for 20 seconds.

- Release the hold and very slowly unroll your spine and return to a sitting position, raising your chest and lengthening your neck as if your head is being pulled gently upward.

- To develop this stretch, once your forehead has touched your knees, gently lower further so that your elbows touch the ground on either side of your knees and hold for 20 seconds before unrolling.

Exercise 77
Lying full body stretch

- Lie flat on your back with legs outstretched and parallel and your arms outstretched and parallel behind your head.

- Breathe out as you point your fingers and toes, stretching them as far away from each other as possible.

- Do not shorten your neck.

- Press your back gently into the floor.

- When you have made yourself as long as possible, hold the stretch for 20 seconds.

- Breathe in and relax.

- Repeat three times.

SPECIFIC SITUATION STRETCHES

The following stretches can be undertaken when you are seated for a long time at your desk, in a car or aeroplane or when using the telephone, to relieve tension and stiffness, boost your energy level and improve circulation. They are sufficient to lubricate the joints with synovial fluid, which will help to prevent or reduce stiffness and reduce wear and tear.

Repeat Exercises 78–91 at regular intervals throughout an air journey to help prevent circulation problems.

Exercise 78
Neck stretch

- Keeping your back straight, very slowly roll your head around in a full circle, stopping to stretch any area that feels tight.

- Slowly stretch your neck upward and back and down so that your chin touches your chest.

- Move the head sideways towards the shoulder, maintaining contact between the chin and the chest throughout the rotation.

- Change direction.

Exercise 79
Forward arm stretch

- Interlace the fingers of both hands and straighten your arms in front of you with palms facing out.

- Feel the stretch in your arms and through the upper part of your back.

- Hold for 20 seconds.

- Repeat three times.

Exercise 80
Upward arm stretch

- Interlace your fingers and turn your palms upwards above your head as you straighten your arms.

- Gently push your hands away from you as far as you can.

- Feel the stretch through your arms and upper sides of your ribcage.

- Hold for 20 seconds.

- Repeat three times.

Exercise 81
Sideways arm stretch

- With your arms extended overhead, hold the outside of your left hand with the right hand and pull your left arm to the side.

- Keep your arms as straight as possible.

- Hold for 20 seconds.

- Repeat on the other side.

Exercise 82
Downwards arm stretch

- Hold your right elbow with your left hand then gently pull it downward behind your head.

- When you feel the stretch in the shoulder and back of the upper arm, hold for 20 seconds.

- Repeat on the other side.

Exercise 83
Forward upper back stretch

- Sit with your right arm straight out in front of you at shoulder height.

- Hold the wrist with your left hand and pull your arm until you feel a stretch in your shoulder.

- Hold for 20 seconds.

- Drop your chin to feel the stretch across your back and hold for 20 seconds.

- Repeat with your left arm.

Exercise 84
Backward upper back stretch

- Interlace your fingers behind your head, keeping your elbows straight out to the side.

- Keep your head and upper body aligned.

- Squeeze your shoulder blades together and when you feel the stretch through your upper back and shoulders, hold for 20 seconds.

- Repeat three times.

Exercise 85
Sideways shoulder stretch

- Hold your right arm just above the elbow with your left hand.

- Gently pull the elbow toward your left shoulder as you look over your right shoulder.

- When you feel the stretch in your shoulder and neck, hold for 20 seconds.

- Repeat on the other side.

Exercise 86
Forearm stretch

■ Place the palms of your hands flat on your chair, level with your hip bones, fingers pointing backwards and thumbs outward.

■ Keeping your palms flat, slowly lean your arms back.

■ When you feel the stretch in your forearms, hold for 20 seconds.

■ Repeat several times.

Exercise 87
Sideways twist

■ With your arms folded in front of you, slowly rotate your body to one side as far as you can, without moving your hips.

■ Allow your head to move with your body.

■ Repeat on the other side.

Exercise 88
Upper leg stretch

■ Hold on to your lower leg just below the knee.

■ Gently pull the knee toward your chest.

■ When you feel a stretch in the side of your upper leg, use the left arm to pull the bent leg across and toward the opposite shoulder.

■ Hold for 20 minutes.

- Repeat with the other side.

Exercise 89
Lower leg stretch

- Straighten your legs in front of you with toes pointed.

- Slowly draw both feet upright and, if you can, towards you.

- When you feel the stretch along the back of your lower leg hold for 20 seconds.

- Release and move your feet away from you, pointing the toes forward as far as you can.

- When you feel the stretch along the front of your legs and in your knees, hold for 20 seconds.

- Relax and repeat three times.

Exercise 90
Ankle stretch

- Rotate each ankle 20 times clockwise and 20 times anticlockwise.

Exercise 91
Forward roll

- Lean forward from your hips, not your waist, downward and towards your toes.

- When you feel the stretch along your spine, hold for 20 seconds.

- Place your hands on your thighs and slowly and gently push the body to an upright position, unrolling vertebra by vertebra.

■ When upright, lengthen your neck as if your head is being gently pulled upwards.

Exercise 92
Telephone stretch

Holding the telephone for a long time causes the neck muscles to stiffen. To avoid stiffness, never cup the phone between ear and shoulder, and change ears often. After the call:

■ Lean your head to the side opposite the ear last used.

■ Lean as far towards the shoulder as possible without straining.

■ When you feel the stretch in your neck, hold for 20 seconds.

■ Repeat on the other side.

Exercise 93
Gridlock stretches (provide a full body workout for when you are stuck in traffic jams)

To stretch the shoulders:

■ Place your hands on the steering wheel at clock position 9.15 with palms facing inward and elbows slightly bent.

■ Slowly move your hands outward as you resist the movement with your shoulder muscles.

■ When you feel the stretch across your shoulders hold for 20 seconds.

- Repeat several times.

For the chest:

- Place your hands on the steering wheel at clock position 9.15, palms facing inwards and elbows slightly bent.

- Push your hands toward each other.

- When you feel the stretch in your chest, hold for 20 seconds.

- Repeat several times.

For the back:

- Hold the steering wheel at clock position 11.05 with outstretched arms and palms facing down.

- Push down on the steering wheel.

- When you feel the stretch in your back, hold for 20 seconds.

- Repeat several times.

For the arms:

- Sit forward in your seat holding your arms bent at right angles close to your body.

- With the palms of your hands facing down and without flexing the head forward, slowly curl your hands up in the direction of your shoulders.

For the abdominals:

- Keeping your body still, stretch your left shoulder towards your left hip.

- Repeat on the other side.

For the buttocks:

- Squeeze your buttocks together as tightly as you can, dimpling them at the sides.

- Hold for 20 seconds.

- Repeat several times.

For the thighs:

- Place your feet flat on the floor hip-width apart.

- Bend your knees at right angles.

- Press both heels downwards until your buttocks are just about to lift off the seat.

- Hold the stretch for 20 seconds.

- Release and repeat several times.

For the lower legs:

- Place one foot flat on the floor and align the knee of the same leg with the heel.

- Place both hands on the knee, palms down and press down.

- Lift your heel rolling the foot onto the ball of the foot.

- When you feel the stretch in your lower leg, hold it for 20 seconds.

- Release and repeat with the other leg.

CHAPTER 7

GETTING A MOVE ON

If you really do want to exercise now is the time to walk your talk. Walking has become the new jogging since studies in the 1990s established that it has similar health and fitness benefits to running. Like running, walking is an aerobic activity. This means that it makes the body demand a greater amount of oxygen by challenging the cardiovascular system (the heart, lungs and circulation) to work harder. Aerobic activity is therefore cardiovascular exercise. It improves cardiovascular efficiency, increases metabolic rate and the production of enzymes that help to burn fat.

THE BENEFITS OF AEROBIC EXERCISE

Regular aerobic exercise has many benefits. It improves heart function, increases the blood supply to the heart and the rest of the body, including the brain, it lowers blood pressure, decreases resting heart rate, increases lung capacity, decreases body fat stores and total cholesterol, reduces tension, symptoms of depression and anxiety, increases energy levels and resistance to fatigue. Regular and frequent aerobic or cardiovascular exercise lowers the risk of coronary heart disease, which kills over 100,000 people in the UK each year. It helps to prevent circulatory and respiratory problems and to control weight. Many experts insist that it is the only way to burn off body fat. Regular aerobic exercise also improves muscle tone and appearance, self-image and self-esteem, mental alertness and the ability to relax.

Accumulating only 30 minutes of aerobic exercise daily will do the trick, and even five minutes a day is better than nothing. To be *really* beneficial, aerobic exercise has to be frequent – meaning at least three times a week. It must last for at least 15 minutes and be hard enough to make you slightly breathless. But you're so relaxed and energised now, you're ready for anything, aren't you?

Aerobic activities include walking, running, cycling, swimming, skiing, rowing, skating, stair climbing – anything that raises your heart rate and increases your oxygen intake.

WALKING

Walking is a highly aerobic activity and one of the best for promoting health and fitness and for reducing the risk of premature death and the onset of dementia in the elderly. Walking also improves mood, with a 10-minute walk having a lasting effect for an hour or more afterwards, and can be equally or more effective than medication in relieving depression. Walking, whether on a treadmill or in the countryside, provides 'time out' from the demands of home and work and can be a very effective anti-stress measure.

Walking is also effective in promoting weight loss, reliably burning calories, with walking a short time after a meal proving to be one of the most effective ways of burning fat, using 15 per cent more calories than walking on an empty stomach. Walking at a steady pace, about 5km per hour, burns calories, but walking uphill (or upstairs) or on softer ground such as grass or sand will burn more. Twenty minutes' fast walking or walking upstairs without stopping (the inspiration for step exercises) will burn more than cycling at that Sunday-afternoon-in-the-sun-out-with-the-family cycling pace you see others doing, and you can use as much energy by walking quickly at 8km per hour as by jogging at the same pace. Amazed? Read on.

Walking is comparable with other aerobic activities in the health benefits it confers but it even has additional advantages. It is a low-impact exercise with low injury potential. It involves nearly all your muscles, not simply those of the legs. The abdominal and back muscles support the spine, head and shoulders and allow the trunk to twist slightly and the arms to work in opposition to the legs. Walking is therefore a full body workout, but this 'walkout' doesn't place much stress on muscles and joints or incur much risk. In contrast, jogging places a lot of strain on the body, particularly on ligaments and joints and isn't suited to those with orthopaedic problems or who are prone to strains and sprains. Jogging also imposes more stress on the cardiovascular system and that can create problems for people with high blood pressure, pulmonary complications or asthma, and those who are overweight.

Walking tones the thighs and buttocks, improves balance, coordination, agility and posture and can contribute to an increase in bone density. As a result it is used by many top athletes and sportsmen and women to complement their training.

It is generally more convenient than many other aerobic activities such as cross-country skiing, rollerblading, rowing or kickboxing and can easily be incorporated into the most sedentary of lifestyles. It's therefore the ideal exercise for the lazy person.

It is the simplest form of exercise. You don't have to learn the skill. It is a physical activity that most people already do. It is easy to do and maintain. It suits all ages and abilities. It can be undertaken by the sick and healthy alike. It can be performed virtually anywhere and at any time. Because it is a simple activity you are more likely to do it more often and for longer than any other form of exercise, so it is easier to accumulate a greater number of 'exercise' sessions per week and consequently achieve better results. The intensity level of this exercise is self-determined. You set your own natural pace and, as fitness develops, increase the pace accordingly and once you feel energised by walking more, the more you will want to walk.

Walking is also the cheapest form of exercise, as it requires no special expensive equipment. Walking is therefore the top choice of aerobic exercise of many fitness coaches, especially for the overweight. Certainly it is the exercise of choice for those wishing to maintain low weight.

Walking is also the form of exercise recommended by most medical practitioners. The noted London-based holistic healthcare practitioner, Dr Mosaraf Ali, strongly advocates walking as exercise for all and regularly takes patients on walking trips to the Himalayas, including those who are seriously ill with chronic fatigue syndrome, ME, nervous disorders, various kinds of paralysis and stress-related conditions. He sums up the health benefits of walking as follows:

It helps to improve blood circulation, it helps to restore joint mobility and reduces joint pain, toxins are eliminated through perspiration, the brain gets fresh oxygen, the digestion is improved, lung capacity and function are improved, it improves posture, it disperses feelings of tiredness and lethargy, walking on green grass improves eyesight, it restores the body's equilibrium, it helps reduce weight, it reduces high blood pressure, it improves skin condition, it reduces stress and tension and it has a beneficial effect on diabetes. Like yoga, it has no age limit. One of the reasons villagers are more healthy than urban dwellers is that they walk a lot. So get out there and walk, walk, walk.

There are countless ways you can build walking, and hence more exercise, into your daily routine. You can walk to work or to the shops, or walk part of the way, getting off the bus or tube a stop before you usually do and walking the remaining distance, or parking further from your destination. You can walk rather than take a taxi and climb stairs rather than take the lift or escalator. Instead of phoning, faxing or e-mailing work colleagues deliver your message personally and benefit from social interaction at the same time. If you must use the phone, pace the floor as you do so, and pace as you think. Instead of having coffee at your desk, walk to the dispenser or café. At lunchtime, take a short walk and 'time out' from the stresses of work or home. Take the children or dog for extra or longer walks. Don't ask others to fetch and carry for you, do things yourself. Dispense with the remote control. By introducing these small changes into your life you will increase the amount of exercise you take, improve fitness and burn calories.

Build short bouts of walking into your day. Longer bouts mean that a person doesn't move around as much as they otherwise might, and will also tend to reward themselves by eating more, which they are less likely to do after a 10-minute activity spurt. Stopping and starting in short but high-intensity bursts of exercise revs up the metabolism and results in positive bodily changes.

If you are ready to use walking as your *primary* exercise, you must ensure that you're walking far enough. You need to walk a minimum of 1.5km (about 2000 steps). You also need to walk aerobically, that is, you must use more oxygen than usual. This means walking briskly rather than merely strolling, at the kind of pace you would use if you were 10 minutes late for an appointment. The difference is that when walking briskly you feel slightly breathless, and although you can hold a conversation, you'd rather not. You can walk aerobically by increasing speed or distance. You can also increase intensity by walking uphill and moving your arms more vigorously. In this way you can make walking an aerobic 'walkout'.

In this chapter there are various exercises which can be incorporated into your walkout, starting with walking and marching on the spot, exercises that can be done anywhere, indoors or out, and which will prepare you for more serious walking. These exercises warm up the legs, mobilise the ankle joints, gently stretch the calf muscles and promote circulation.

Exercise 94
Walking on the spot

- Get comfortable. Stand upright as if strings attached to your head are pulling you gently upwards lengthening your neck and the spine along its length.

- Keep your shoulders down in your back.

- Relax your chest.

- Allow your arms to fall by your sides with your elbows slightly away from your body.

- Align your pelvis with your head.

- Stand with your feet hip-width apart and your weight evenly on both feet. Don't allow them to roll inward or outward.

- Breathing normally, rise up onto the balls of your feet, ensuring that your body doesn't pitch forward.

- Lower your left heel to the ground, bending your right knee directly over the centre of your right foot as you do so.

- Swap legs so that you are walking on the spot.

- Repeat 50 times, keeping your body length and your weight centred.

- Don't wiggle your hips. Keep your pelvis level throughout.

Exercise 95
Marching on the spot with biceps curl

In addition to warming up the legs, this strengthens and shapes the biceps, the front of the arms and shoulders.

- Stand upright, your feet hip-width apart.

- March on the spot.

- As you raise each knee, swing the opposite arm with loosely clenched fist turned uppermost towards your shoulder.

- Increase the intensity by raising your knees higher and

clenching your fists more tightly.

- Increase the pace and continue for two minutes.

- To further tone the muscles of the upper legs, march with feet wider than hip-width apart for two minutes.

- For one minute alternate marching wide and with feet hip-width apart.

WALKING OUT

Before attempting the following exercises ensure that you read the guidelines below on technique. Irrespective of how far or quickly you walk, you must ensure that you walk correctly.

Walking technique

It is important to keep your head up and your neck relaxed when walking. Research has shown that walkers who keep their eyes focused on the horizon use more calories than those who look down at the ground! Looking down also puts pressure on your neck and spine. Keep your shoulders up and level rather than hunched, and your back straight. Keep your arms close to your body and swing them forward at waist height to propel yourself forward. Your hips should be in line with your shoulders and they should rotate from front to back with each stride and not side to side. Don't waddle or exaggerate your hip movements. And don't overstride by taking longer steps in front of your body. Your stride should be longer behind your body than in front so the force of the stride comes from pushing off your back foot and engaging the hamstring muscles at the back of your thighs and the gluteal muscles of your buttocks. Always push off forcefully from the toe of the foot behind the body and strike the ground noiselessly with your heel and your ankle flexed so that someone standing in front should be able to see the entire sole of your foot with every step. Roll through the step from the heel to the ball of the foot. To add speed increase the number of strides you take rather than lengthening your stride. Breathe rhythmically through your mouth.

It is not advisable to wear walking shoes designed for hiking. These offer the stability and support essential for rough terrain but they are not flexible enough to allow your foot to roll in the way that is required for fast walking. Cross-training shoes or running shoes are more suitable.

Exercise 96
Progressive walkout

This can be performed as a progressive series of exercises, or, when fitness increases, as one exercise. To progress, start by walking three times a week building up to five times a week within a month. Aim to increase your pace by decreasing the number of minutes you take to walk a kilometre. Start by walking 1.5km in 20 minutes and aim to reduce this to 15 minutes within six weeks. Each week add five minutes to each walk so that you start by walking for 15 minutes and by week seven you are walking for 50 minutes.

Level 1
Allow 16–20 minutes for 1.5km.

- Walk with your posture upright, head up and looking directly ahead.

- Allow your arms to swing from the shoulder.

- Maintain a comfortable length of stride.

Level 2

Increase your speed to 13–15 minutes per 1.5km.

- Use your arms more forcefully, keeping them flexed at 90 degrees at the elbows. Don't swing the arms across your body.

- On the forward swing the arms shouldn't swing higher than your chest.

- On the backward swing, push your elbows back so that your hands are almost at hip level but don't let the hands go behind your hips.

- Fully extend the back leg but don't lock the knee as this will cause you strain the knee. Don't over-bend the knee as this will cause you to bob up and down.

- Allow the hips to move forward and back naturally.

- As you increase your speed you will tend to lean forward slightly. Ensure that this begins from the ankle and not the waist.

Level 3

Increase your speed to 12 minutes per 1.5km or faster.

- Don't allow yourself to wiggle as your hip action becomes more pronounced.

- Cool down by returning gradually to a steady walking pace.

- Stretch (see calf, thigh and hamstring stretches on pages

72–5) and to prevent muscle soreness.

Exercise 97
Power walking

Aim to walk at 10 minutes per 1.5km.

■ Focus on pushing off through the back leg and ensuring that the toe of that leg leaves the ground last.

■ Keep your head and chest up.

■ Hold in the muscles of the abdomen.

■ Squeeze the buttock of the leg that is behind with each stride.

■ Breathe rhythmically through the mouth.

■ After power walking, don't forget to cool down and stretch (see calf, thigh and hamstring stretches pages 72–5) to prevent muscle soreness.

This is a demanding exercise and you may experience discomfort in the front of your legs from below the knees to the ankles if your shin muscles are unaccustomed to vigorous exercise. This will diminish over time as your muscles strengthen but it may help to begin every walk by toe tapping each foot. To do these simply plant your foot on the ground and raise and lower the foot 30–50 times. You can also strengthen your shin muscles by walking around the house on your heels whenever you can.

Interval training walkout

An excellent cardiovascular exercise is to alternate fast walking with walking at a slower moderate pace. This effectively kick starts and revs the cardiovascular system. You can use lampposts or telegraph poles as a measure of the intervals for each phase of the exercise. Remember to cool down at the end of the exercise.

UP AND RUNNING

When walking fast or power walking you may find that you want to break into a slow jog (a pace between walking and running) or a faster run. You may even find it difficult not to do so. However, don't rush to do so. Progress at your own pace, and if and when you do begin to jog remember to remain unhurried and relaxed. Avoid carrying unnecessary tension, especially in the shoulders.

If you feel inclined to run, especially on a regular basis, ensure that you are wearing shoes that provide adequate support for your heels and the arches of your feet and also some cushioning against the concussion involved. Purpose-designed running shoes are ideal. You will probably find that you need to wear much looser and lighter clothing than when simply walking, so running is likely to run up additional costs.

It is not necessary to go for a run to derive some of the benefits of running. Jogging on the spot is an excellent and simple cardiovascular exercise. For this reason it is usually included in any warm-up prior to vigorous exercise.

Exercise 98
Jogging on the spot with biceps curl

■ Keep an upright body posture with head up and eyes looking straight ahead.

■ Run on the spot, bringing your heels up towards the backs of your knees, making sure that with each step you place the heel on the ground.

■ Relax your shoulders.

■ Keep your arms close in to the sides of your body, elbows bent at 90 degrees and loosely clenched fists turned upward, alternately raise each arm towards the shoulders.

■ Continue for 1–5 minutes.

■ To increase intensity jog faster.

■ Do not let your head drop or your neck shorten.

Exercise 99
Jogging with legs wide apart and biceps curl

To vary the above exercise and tone the outer thighs and calf muscles, jog on the spot with the feet wider than hip-width apart. Make sure you lower the heel to the ground on each step. Alternate 30-second intervals of jogging in this way with 30-second intervals or ordinary jogging on the spot.

Exercise 100
Sprinting on the spot

This exercise is effective in quickly raising heart and breathing rates.

■ Keep an upright posture and stand with feet hip-width apart.

■ Begin by jogging on the spot slowly.

■ Increase the pace until you are running on the spot as fast as you can.

- Use your arms as pistons to power the action.

- Lower the heels to the floor with each step.

- As you run faster you will tend to lean forward slightly. Make sure you are leaning from the ankle, not from the waist.

- Try not to look down and/or hunch the shoulders forward.

- Continue for 30 seconds.

- Jog on the spot at normal pace for 30 seconds.

- Alternate sprinting and jogging in 30-second intervals for five minutes.

If you'd rather not *go out* walking and measuring speeds and distances, you may find a treadmill useful. These machines can be used for walking or running and can be set for specific distances and speed. Some have heart monitors so that you can check your heart rate as you exercise and most have calorie meters so that you can see how much energy you are using. Some have an incline option that tilts the treadmill, producing inclines of varying degrees to simulate hill walking. The intensity of a treadmill walkout can be increased as fitness improves. To use a treadmill to warm up, five minutes walking or jogging is adequate. For a full cardiovascular workout 20 minutes is the recommended minimum. Remember that walking at 4.5km per hour is as effective as jogging at the same speed. However, while walking on a treadmill may seem like an easy option, it is not: the pace doesn't slacken and if you don't keep up you fall off the machine!

Exercise 101
Treadmill walkout

Stand tall, keep your posture upright and look straight ahead. Don't hunch your back and shoulders.

- Walk steadily with a heel-to-toe action. Don't walk on your toes.

- Relax your shoulders and swing your arms freely as you walk.

- Keep your chest and breathing relaxed.

- Warm up at a slow comfortable pace for up to five minutes then increase to a demanding pace that makes you slightly breathless, continuing for 20 minutes.

- Cool down by slowing to a slow pace for up to five minutes.

The advantages of using a treadmill are that it can be used in all weathers, you avoid breathing in polluted air and it prevents the need to walk outdoors after dark. The drawback is that it is an expensive and space-consuming piece of equipment, so unless you have plenty of money and space to spare or are willing to go to a gym you are probably better off walking to work every day.

However, at this stage you may want to proceed to other cardiovascular exercise. If you are feeling the benefits of relaxation, stretching and walking you may want to try aerobic or step aerobic classes. If you can't afford or don't want to pay for gym classes you can easily do this kind of exercise at home. Aerobic exercise is, as we have seen, anything that increases the heart rate and makes you slightly breathless. Walking and jogging on the spot to music are the basis of most aerobic exercise classes.

Various dance steps and movements are added to increase intensity and add variety. You can improvise your own programme or borrow exercise videos from your local library and benefit from many different instructors and styles of exercise until you find ones that suit you best.

Step aerobics involves stepping up and down off a low platform to music. It impacts on the body in much the same way as walking but can be as intense as running. You can buy an exercise step, but you can get similar benefits from climbing stairs continually for a given period, or using just the bottom stair to step up and down. Learn a few step moves and techniques from books or videos.

Now that you are feeling some of the benefits of exercise – no doubt feeling better for being more active *and* enjoying it – you might be thinking seriously about 'taking the next step'. Chapter 8, Going Further, will tell you all you need to know about going to a gym.

CHAPTER 8

GOING FURTHER

Fitness means different things to different people. To some it means not simply being without the symptoms of illness, but being healthy, feeling well and having abundant energy. For others it may mean fitness to perform specific activities or skills, whether that is climbing stairs, tying shoelaces, mowing the lawn, running a marathon or competing in an Olympic triathlon. You may see it as a combination of both. Whatever your definition, you can benefit from leading a more active life and by so doing increasing your level of personal fitness. Though physical fitness is not in itself equivalent with health and well-being, it makes an important contribution to both.

There are several elements to health-related physical fitness (as opposed to skill-related fitness) and these are: body composition, cardiovascular endurance, flexibility, muscular endurance and muscular strength:

Body composition is the ratio of body fat to lean body tissue – as opposed to body weight. It determines the level of fat in the body, which is an important factor in health.

Cardiovascular endurance or aerobic fitness is the ability to maintain a moderate level of activity using the large muscles of the body (as in walking, running or swimming) for a minimum period of time (15–20 minutes) – long enough to produce beneficial changes to the heart, lungs and circulatory system.

Flexibility is the range of movement in each of the joints, enabling you to perform everyday activities safely and efficiently.

Muscular endurance is the capacity for a muscle or group of muscles to maintain or repeat a movement for a set period of time without getting tired.

Muscular strength is the amount of force exerted by a muscle or group of muscles – meaning how much weight you can lift or push.

These components can all be trained to some degree and so can be improved by a certain amount of regular exercise. A balanced exercise programme aimed at improving all-round fitness should include all the health-related fitness components. The relaxation, breathing, stretching and cardiovascular exercises in this book will help you to improve flexibility, cardiovascular endurance and body composition. However, exercises that improve flexibility and cardiovascular functioning are not necessarily effective for developing muscular strength and endurance. To do this, *resistance training* is needed. That means working with weights to create resistance against which the muscles of the body work in the action of lifting or pushing. This tones and strengthens the muscles of the body, including the heart, which is a muscle. Resistance training therefore has cardiovascular benefits. It also strengthens joints helping to prevent injury, builds bone density and burns calories and is effective in preventing many of the problems associated with ageing, such as joint problems, osteoporosis and weight gain.

WEIGHTY ISSUES

There are several myths about training with weights that deter many people, especially women, from attempting it.

Brawn equals bulk

A common misconception is that exercising with weights builds huge muscles in women but this is only achieved by working with enormous weights for hours every day. Lifting light weights helps build a more natural toned body shape. Many top athletes and sportsmen and women, including golfers and tennis players, train with weights to help improve sports performance while remaining slender.

Training with weights for 25-minutes two to three times weekly yields dramatic results. It's possible to add 1.5kg of muscle in a week, while losing 1–3kg of fat without changing your eating habits. The importance of increasing muscle is that it burns 35–50 calories for every 0.5kg of body weight per day simply sustaining itself. The more muscle mass in your body the higher your metabolic rate will be and the more efficient your body will be at burning fat. So, the more muscle you have the more fat you will burn when you are inactive. This is because your resting metabolic rate – the rate at which calories are burned at rest – is closely linked to muscle mass. Ultimately, it is not the calories burned during exercise that are important but those burned when you're not active. Loss of muscle slows down the resting metabolic rate and so fewer calories are burned. You can benefit from working with weights as little as 10 minutes four or five times weekly.

Brawn becomes blubber

Another widely held misconception is that muscle developed by exercise will turn to fat if exercise is stopped. However, muscle and fat are two completely different substances and one doesn't convert into the other. It is only loss of condition that alters the appearance of the body.

Going to the gym makes you slim

It is generally true that, in relation to weight training, gyms and fitness centres have many advantages. They usually provide a wide range of equipment for both aerobic exercise and resistance training, and exercise programmes, such as circuit training and body pump, that combine both types of exercise. However, in some cases going to the gym may not help you to lose weight and may even make you put it on.

Many of those who regularly work out at the gym tend to reward themselves between sessions by eating more and lying on the sofa watching television. As a result they burn fewer calories in total than those who don't go to the gym at all but lead a moderately active life by walking or cycling regularly. But to make things worse, the calorie metres on most pieces of gym equipment are often an unreliable guide to calories burned as they give only an approximate average reading. Those using them can be led to believe they are working off more calories than they actually are.

Many people use their exercise sessions to cancel out overeating or excessive drinking at other times. This 'pay back' approach to exercise is singularly unsuccessful. If you exercise four hours a week in a gym, 164 hours of the week remain – those hours are the important ones. There is little point spending 20 minutes exercising on a stepper machine in a gym if you habitually take escalators and in lifts rather than climb stairs, or drive a short distance to the gym to walk on a treadmill. Just remaining on your feet most of the day rather than being sedentary will increase the calories you burn.

This is not to say that there's no point in joining a gym. There are many benefits to be gained from a formal or structured exercise routine that you don't get simply from being more active. However, if you've come this far and still hate the idea of attending a gym, don't worry, and don't give up on the idea of exercise, especially if you are trying to lose weight. You can undertake a formal and structured resistance exercise routine at home.

What you'll need is two pairs of hand-held weights of 1–5kg. Make your own by filling plastic bottles with sand, or invest in a couple of pairs of vinyl-covered dumbbells (1 and 2–2.5kg or 2–2.5 and 5kg depending on your size and strength). You can even train without weights once you understand the correct movement and can work the muscles correctly.

GUIDELINES FOR RESISTANCE TRAINING

- Always stretch beforehand in order to warm up your muscles, increase your heart rate and circulation and avoid injury. The following stretches are recommended before working with weights: calf stretches, thigh stretch, hamstring stretch, lower back stretch, overhead side bends, scapular squeeze, shoulder and upper back stretches, chest and arm stretches, head rolls (see Chapter 6).

- Start all exercises by standing with your feet shoulder-width apart.

- Keep your head up, chin level and eyes looking straight ahead. Do not arch your back or hunch your shoulders.

- Keep your knees soft (not locked).

- Use light weights.

- Lift the weights with controlled movements. Do not jerk them.

- Breathe out on the exertion and breathe in when returning to the start position.

- Tighten your abdominal muscles during the lift to support your back.

- Initially perform 10 repetitions of each exercise and as you improve, two sets of 10 repetitions, progressing to three sets of each, and resting between each set.

- Gradually increase the number of repetitions to 12–15.

- When the exercise becomes too easy increase the weights used.

- Start by exercising the larger muscle groups of your body when your energy level is highest, working down to the smaller muscle groups where less energy is required. Follow this order: chest, back, thighs; shoulders, biceps, triceps, calves and forearms.

- Never continue to work if you feel dizzy, fatigued or suspect that you have strained a muscle.

- Always cool down by stretching to relax your muscles and prevent muscle soreness.

Exercise 102
Flyes

Works the chest and front of the shoulder.

■ Lie on the floor or a bench (if on the floor bend your knees and place your feet flat on the floor hip-width apart).

■ Hold a dumbbell in each hand, directly above your chest,

palms facing each other and the dumbbells touching.

- Keep your elbows slightly bent.

- Breathe out and open your arms until your arms are parallel to the floor. Hold briefly.

- Breathe in as you return to the start position.

- Repeat 10 times.

Exercise 103
Side lateral raise

Works the shoulders.

- Stand as instructed above with your feet firmly on the floor or sit on a chair holding a dumbbell in each hand with palms facing your sides, arms relaxed and straight. Do not bend your wrists.

- Keep your back straight.

- With arms straight but elbows not locked, raise both dumbbells straight up to the side until they reach shoulder height, breathing out as you do so.

- Hold this position briefly before slowly lowering your arms to the start position, breathing in as you do so.

- Repeat 10 times.

Exercise 104
Side bends

Works the outer abdominal muscles.

- Stand with feet shoulder-width apart.

- Hold a dumbbell in each hand.

- Keeping your neck straight, breathe in and bend to one side as far as you can.

- Hold the position briefly then breathe out as you return to the start position.

- Repeat 10 times on each side.

Exercise 105
Front shoulder lift

Works the chest and front of the shoulders.

- Stand with your feet shoulder-width apart and knees slightly bent.

- Keep your back straight and not arched.

- Hold a dumbbell in each hand with palms facing down towards the front of your body.

- Breathe out as you raise your right arm in the air in front of your body until the weight is at shoulder height.

- Hold the position briefly.

- Breathe in as you slowly lower your arm to the start position.

- Raise your left arm and repeat 10 times with each arm.

Exercise 106
Biceps curl

Works the biceps.

- Stand with your feet shoulder-width apart, hips tucked in and shoulders dropped and relaxed, a dumbbell in each hand in front of your body with palms facing forward, resting against your thighs.

■ Keep your back straight (you can stand with your back pressed against a wall to help ensure this).

■ Bending from the elbow only, bring the dumbbell in your right hand upward until it touches the front of your chest. Control the movement. Do not swing the dumbbell. Keep your elbows close to your body.

■ Breathe out as you raise the dumbbell toward you.

■ Slowly breathe in as you return to the start position.

This exercise can be performed with a barbell – a metal bar with weights at each end – in order to work both arms at the same time.

Exercise 107
Overhead extension

Works the triceps.

■ Sit on a chair or bench with your back straight, chin up and looking straight ahead. Don't arch your back.

■ Hold a single dumbbell in both hands behind your head with palms facing upwards.

■ Keep your upper arms close to your head.

■ Bend your arms at the elbows.

■ Breathe in as you slowly lower the dumbbell as far as you can behind your neck.

- Hold the position briefly, then breathe out and slowly straighten your arms above your head.

- Repeat 10 times.

Exercise 108
Side squats

Works the front and back of the thighs and the buttocks.

- Stand with feet apart, toes pointing outward.

- Hold a dumbbell in each hand at hip height.

- Breathe in as you slowly lower your body until your thighs are parallel with the floor.

- Hold the position and then tighten your buttocks and slowly return to the start position.

- Repeat 10 times.

Exercise 109
Forward lunges

Works the thighs and buttocks.

- Stand with your feet shoulder-width apart and your back straight.

- Keep your hips square to the floor.

- Hold dumbbells in each hand at hip height with arms relaxed and elbows not locked.

- Breathe in and take a long step forward, keeping the weight of your body centred over your hips, your body straight and your foot in line with your hips.

■ Hold before breathing out and slowly returning to the start position.

■ Repeat 10 times with each leg.

Exercise 110
Shoulder press

Works the shoulders.

■ Sit on a chair or bench with a dumbbell in each hand, your back straight and feet flat on the floor.

■ Bend your elbows and hold the dumbbells at shoulder height close to your body with your palms facing forward.

■ Breathe out as you press the dumbbells straight up to arm length.

■ Breathe out as you return to the starting position.

■ Repeat 10 times.

Exercise 111
Abdominal stretch

Works the muscles of the abdomen.

■ Lie on the floor or a bench (if on the floor lie with knees bent and both feet flat on the floor hip-width apart) holding a single dumbbell in both hands at arm's length above your head.

■ Breathe out and slowly lower the dumbbell behind your head so that it is in line with your body.

■ Do not allow your back to arch.

- Hold, breathe in and slowly return to the start position.

- Repeat 10 times.

For the following exercises you will require ankle weights – cuffs containing weights held in place by adjustable Velcro straps. These can be bought from a sports shop. You can make your own by filling the middle section of a nylon stocking with dried rice, knotting both ends to form an anklet, and cutting the remaining stocking so that you leave ties on each end.

Exercise 112
Rear knee lift

Works the thighs and buttocks.

- Attach ankle weights to each ankle and lower yourself onto all fours.

- Breathe in and lift your right leg behind you until your thigh is parallel with the floor. Do not lift the leg higher than this.

- Keep your head and spine straight, holding your abdominal muscles tight to help support your back.

- Breathe out as you return to the start position.

- Repeat 10 times with each leg.

Exercise 113
Leg curl

Works the back of the thighs, the inner thighs and the sides of the lower leg.

- Wearing leg weights, stand with your feet together and place your hands on the back of a chair for support.

- Bend one knee until the lower leg is parallel to the floor.

- Keep your thighs straight and do not move your upper leg.

- Keep your buttocks tight to support the lower back.

- Breathe in and slowly lower your foot to the floor.

- Slowly breathe out and bring your foot back up until your leg is once again parallel to the floor.

- Repeat 10 times with each leg.

Exercise 114
Inner thigh lifts

Works the inner thighs.

- Wearing ankle weights, lie on the floor on your right side with your back straight, hips square and feet together.

- Support your head in your right hand and place your left hand in front of your body for balance.

- Ensure that your right leg is straight and bend your left leg at a right angle to your body for support.

- Breathe out as you slowly raise your right leg as high as possible.

- Hold briefly and breathe in as you lower your leg.

- Repeat 10 times with each leg.

Exercise 115
Outer thigh stretch

Works the outer thigh.

- Wearing leg weights, lie on your right side in a straight line. Stretch out your right arm in line with your body and rest your head on it. Keep your waist off the floor.

- Bend both legs in front of you at 90 degrees.

- Place your left arm in front of your body for balance.

- Tighten your abdominal muscles, breathe out and take the top leg back in line with your hip about 12cms from the floor, flexing the foot towards your face.

- Breathe out and slowly raise the leg about 15cms.

- Hold briefly before breathing in and lowering the leg.

- Repeat 10 times with each leg.

GETTING THERE

The exercises in this chapter provide a full body, resistance training programme. Ideally the programme should be incorporated into a fitness regime that includes stretching and cardiovascular exercise. Twenty minutes of each three times a week will yield noticeable health and fitness benefits after as little as three weeks. If you accomplish this, you certainly won't be lazy any more. And you might even be ready to consider joining a gym.

So, what can you expect?

A good gym or fitness centre will be clean and orderly and its staff will show you the facilities on offer without any obligation to join. It will have a range of equipment: cardiovascular machines, such as various kinds of exercise bike, rowing machines, treadmills, versa climbers (to simulate mountain climbing), steppers and cross-trainers (to simulate cross-country skiing); resistance training equipment such as free weights (dumbbells and barbells); and machines such as a pec deck, a leg curler, bench press and leg press. The equipment should all be well maintained. Details of qualified staff and persons trained in first aid, both of whom should be available at all times, will be posted on notice boards.

As a prospective member you'll be asked to complete a simple health-screening questionnaire to establish any medical conditions and family health history to ensure you're not at risk and you'll be asked to undertake an assessment to determine your level of fitness before a suitable programme of exercise is planned. This could involve tests to establish your resting heart rate and a cycle test to indicate your current level of fitness. A body fat test using a simple instrument that calculates body fat index may also be included. After this simple procedure a qualified instructor will demonstrate the use of the equipment and answer any questions you have. You will also be given details of the classes and activities scheduled at the gym and the different membership schemes. If you decide to join the gym you'll have a fitness programme tailored to your own fitness requirements and it will be updated by appropriate staff as your fitness improves. And the fitter – and more relaxed – you become, the less lazy you will feel. Just ask anyone at the gym!

BIBLIOGRAPHY

Brown, J.D. (1991) 'Staying fit and staying well: physical fitness as a moderator of life stress', *Journal of Personality and Social Psychology*, 60, 4, 555–61.

Brown, J.D. and J.M. Siegel (1988) 'Exercise as a buffer of life stress: a prospective study of adolescents', *Health Psychology*, 7, 553–68.

Brown, S. (2001) 'Do workouts make you fat?', *Sunday Times*. 8 April.

Cousins, N. (1981) *Anatomy of an illness as perceived by the patient; reflections on healing and regeneration*. New York: Bantam Books.

Dostalek, C. (1987) 'The empirical and experimental foundation of Yoga Therapy' in Gharote, .M.I. and M. Lockhart, *The Art of Survival: A guide to yoga therapy*. London: Unwin Hyman Ltd.

Gosselin, C. (1995) *The Ultimate Guide to Fitness*. London: Vermillion.

Hendler, S.S.H. (1989) *The Oxygen Breakthrough*. New York: Morrow Books.

Holmes, D.S. and D.L. Roth (1985) 'Association of aerobic fitness with pulse rate and subjective responses to psychological stress', *Psychophysiology*, 22, 525–9.

Keller, S. & P. Seraganian (1984) 'Physical fitness level and autonomic reactivity to stress', *Journal of Psychosomatic Research*, 28, 279–87.

Light, K.C. et al. (1987) 'Cardiovascular responses to stress II. Relationships to aerobic exercise patterns', *Psychophysiology*, 24, 79–86.

Mosaraf A. (2001) *The Integrated Health Bible*. London: Vermilion Ebury Press.

Phillimore, J. (2001) 'Why we all hate exercise', *You* magazine. *Mail on Sunday,* 31 December.

Rodin, J. (1986) 'Aging and health: effects of the sense of control', *Science*, 232, 1271–6.

Rogers, L. (2001) 'Medical Notes', *Sunday Times,* Style, 1 April.

Shaw, W.A. (1946) 'The relaxation of muscular action potentials to imaginal weightlifting', *Archives of Psychology*, 247, 250.

Simons, A.D. et al. (1985) 'Exercise as a treatment for depression: an update', *Clinical Psychology Review*, 5, 553–68.

Sinyor, D. et al. (1986) 'Experimental manipulation of aerobic fitness and the response to psychosocial stress: heart rate and self report measures', *Psychosomatic Medicine*, 48, 324–37.

Wadud, Swami Deva (undated) *Osho Meditation. The first and last freedom. A practical guide to meditation*, 4th edition. Osho International Foundation. Rebel Publishing House.

Waterman, N. cited Shabi. R. (2001) 'Short cuts', *Sunday Times,* Style, 25 February.

SHERRY FITZGERALD.

062 - 63743.

Killenaule 3 Bed DETACHED.

€150 - 000

Glengoole South